SHOPPER

SUPERMARKET SHOPPER

The Guide to Healthy Eating

Dr Trevor Smith

MAINSTREAM PUBLISHING

EDINBURGH AND LONDON

First published in Great Britain in 1996 by
MAINSTREAM PUBLISHING COMPANY (EDINBURGH) LTD
7 Albany Street
Edinburgh EH1 3UG

ISBN 1 85158 792 6

A catalogue recordfor this book is available from the British Library

Typeset in Palatino
Printed and bound by WSOY, Finland

This book is dedicated to my parents who always made me eat my greens, to my wife, Janette, who always eats hers, and to our son, David, whom we are still trying to persuade to eat his.

Acknowledgements

Thanks are due to the countless numbers of researchers who, over the years, have painstakingly analysed our diet and discovered what the main nutrients are, why we need them, and what foods they are to be found in, so that people like us can build up a picture of what constitutes a healthy diet. Thanks also to the numerous relatives, friends and acquaintances whose eating patterns, both good and bad, have inspired this book. For his great care in typing and retyping the manuscript, I have only myself to thank, as I can't afford a typist.

Contents

MEDICAL NOTE

This book is intended for everyone, young or not so young who wants to adopt a healthy diet. However if you have any problems such as diabetes or heart disease, or are pregnant or grossly over- or under-weight, you should seek the advice of your family doctor as well.

CHAPTER 1

Introduction

Healthy eating should be fun, but there is a serious side too, so let us get that over in the first page or so, and then we will be free to enjoy our conducted tour of the local supermarket.

Premature deaths from heart disease in Britain are amongst the highest in the world, and the high-fat British diet must share the blame. The average British diet is one of the worst in the developed world. We eat far too little fruit and vegetables and far too much saturated fat. The World Health Organisation recommends that we should obtain no more than 10 per cent of our energy from saturated fat, yet in Britain it currently contributes 16 per cent. At least half of our energy should be obtained instead from the starch of cereals and vegetables.

Two recent government reports – the 1994 *COMA Report* for the whole of the UK and *The Scottish Diet* for north of the border – have presented further evidence of the inadequacies of our diet and made recommendations as to what changes need to be made. Those of us living in the areas of Britain with the worst diets are advised to:

1 Double the amount of fresh fruit we eat.
2 Double the amount of fresh and frozen vegetables we eat.
3 Increase the bread we eat by half with wholemeal bread.

4 Double the breakfast cereals we eat.
5 Reduce the processed meat and sausages we eat by half.
6 Replace all of the whole (full fat) milk we drink by semi-skimmed, except for children under two years.
7 Reduce the butter we eat by two-thirds.
8 Double the amount of oily fish we eat.
9 Reduce the cakes, biscuits and pastry we eat by half.
10 Reduce the amount of confectionery, soft drinks and savoury snacks by a third for adults and a half for children.
11 Reduce the sugar and preserves we eat by half.

These are overall targets and as individuals, whether we need to double, quadruple, reduce by a half, or keep at the same level, our consumption of a particular kind of food will obviously depend on how much of it we eat at the moment. By always choosing the healthy, low fat option, we may not need to reduce the amount of a particular product at all. The overall recommendations, however, provide an excellent guide as to what current medical opinion considers to be the healthiest foods that we should be eating most of and the not so healthy that we should only eat occasionally.

The aim of this book is to help you choose from the produce on sale at your local supermarket, town centre or corner shop, which are the best buys. Out of a dozen brands of breakfast cereal or baked beans some will be healthier than others. How do we choose the healthy option? Meat can be a healthy source of first-class protein or a slab of deadly saturated fat depending on what animal it comes from. How do we choose? Which are the healthy fats and which are the harmful and where are the different kinds found? Which are the best kinds of fish to buy? Which dairy products can we continue to enjoy and

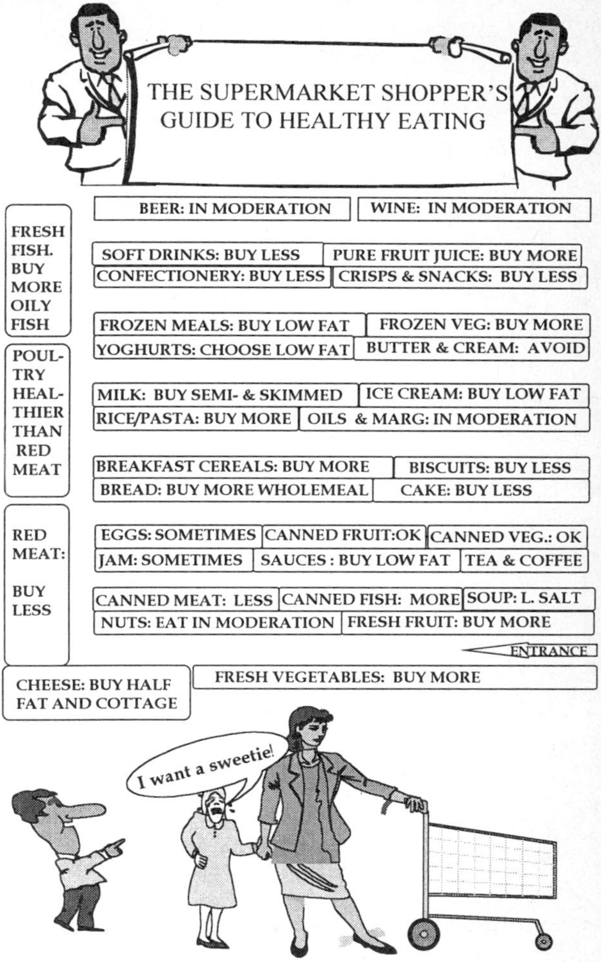
THE SUPERMARKET SHOPPER'S GUIDE TO HEALTHY EATING
BEER: IN MODERATION
WINE: IN MODERATION
FRESH FISH. BUY MORE OILY FISH
SOFT DRINKS: BUY LESS
PURE FRUIT JUICE: BUY MORE
CONFECTIONERY: BUY LESS
CRISPS & SNACKS: BUY LESS
FROZEN MEALS: BUY LOW FAT
FROZEN VEG: BUY MORE
YOGHURTS: CHOOSE LOW FAT
BUTTER & CREAM: AVOID
POULTRY HEALTHIER THAN RED MEAT
MILK: BUY SEMI- & SKIMMED
ICE CREAM: BUY LOW FAT
RICE/PASTA: BUY MORE
OILS & MARG: IN MODERATION
BREAKFAST CEREALS: BUY MORE
BISCUITS: BUY LESS
BREAD: BUY MORE WHOLEMEAL
CAKE: BUY LESS
CHECKOUTS
RED MEAT: BUY LESS
EGGS: SOMETIMES
CANNED FRUIT:OK
CANNED VEG.: OK
JAM: SOMETIMES
SAUCES : BUY LOW FAT
TEA & COFFEE
CANNED MEAT: LESS
CANNED FISH: MORE
SOUP: L. SALT
NUTS: EAT IN MODERATION
FRESH FRUIT: BUY MORE
ENTRANCE
CHEESE: BUY HALF FAT AND COTTAGE
FRESH VEGETABLES: BUY MORE
I want a sweetie!

which should we avoid? Why is excessive consumption of cakes and biscuits so bad for us? Should we give up eating eggs because of fears about cholesterol? What vitamins and minerals do we need, why do we need them and what kinds of food are they found in?

The *Supermarket Shopper* provides an answer to these questions and many, many more. It advises us to 'Read That Label' and shows us what to look out for. Once we have grasped a few simple principles and acquired some skill in label reading, selecting the Healthy Option soon becomes a matter of course.

CHAPTER 2

The Fresh Fruit Section

Official Recommendation: We should (as a population) double the amount of fresh fruit we eat.

FRUIT FOR NATURAL SUGAR, FIBRE, VITAMINS AND MINERALS

Let us make an imaginary visit to our favourite supermarket and see what's on offer. Is any of it worth eating? Let's collect a trolley from the entrance and I'll lead the charge into the supermarket through the automatic doors. One of these days those doors aren't going to open and I'm going to end up with a trolley full of glass!

Our journey through the typical supermarket starts with the fruit and vegetable section. This is the place to come when we want a quick snack or dessert! Most people in Britain eat far too little fruit. It is recommended that: *Everyone should aim to eat at least three pieces of fruit the size of an apple or banana every day.*

Yet in a recent Health Survey carried out on behalf of the Department of Health, no less than one in three of the 16,000 people questioned revealed that they eat fresh fruit less than three times a week, let alone three times a day! It was a bit more encouraging to find that half of those questioned eat fruit once a day, but only one in five said they did so *more* than once a day. We clearly have a long way to go to achieve the healthy Mediterranean diet where fresh fruit is eaten at virtually every meal and in between meals.

Apples

Near the entrance are the fruits that some of us grow in our own gardens. Let's take a look first at the apples. This is the fruit you really can eat between meals without ruining your appetite. Tear off a plastic bag and start collecting! One of Britain's most popular apples is Cox's Orange Pippin. It tastes good but is low in vitamin C. Sturmer Pippin has six times as much! Home grown apples are supplemented with other varieties imported from France, the United States and New Zealand to make sure we can partake of our apple a day every day of the year.

Here's the first tip. As different varieties of apple vary so much in the amount of the vitamins and minerals they contain, to get the most that they have to offer, get into the habit of buying lots of different varieties rather than sticking to the same one all of the time. The same principle applies to all fruit and vegetables. Eat a variety of varieties!

Pears

As with apples there are both dessert and cooking varieties of pears but virtually all of those offered for sale in the supermarket are dessert types. Although there are hundreds of varieties, most supermarkets typically stock Conference and Comice and possibly William's so our choice tends to be more limited than with apples. Pears have the annoying habit of taking a long time to get ripe and juicy and then going off quickly once they are ripe, but you can control the process to some extent with temperature. Putting them in a warm spot encourages ripening and once ripe the deterioration can be delayed for a few days by placing them in the refrigerator.

Plums
Choose plums which are firm and have a distinct bloom on the surface. If it's a rich, sweet flavour you are looking for, try the round, red Santa rosa and the round, violet Kirke's Blue. The Victoria and Japanese plums in contrast are rather bland. Several varieties of plum are dried to produce prunes.

Peaches and Apricots
Peaches may have white or yellow skins. The white-skinned varieties are generally considered sweeter. If we are not ready to eat them immediately they can be kept for several days in the refrigerator. To make peaches easier to peel pop them in boiling water for a few seconds. Fresh peaches have about five times as much vitamin C as the canned varieties which most of us tend to eat more of.

Apricots look like small peaches. Choose the ones with the least wrinkled and darkest skins. If necessary, they can be ripened by leaving them in a warm room for a day or two. As with peaches, the skin can be removed most easily if they are plunged into boiling water for a few seconds. There are many uses for apricots apart from eating them fresh. Some cooks stew them, poach them for serving with chicken, fill pies with them, or turn them into jam or even wine.

Melons
Another excellent fruit. Although the shape of the Honeydew and Lavan melons may appeal to the rugby supporter, their tough skins make it difficult to tell if they are ripe or not. The smaller, rounder Charantais, Ogen

and especially the Cantaloupe melons generally have a sweeter, more fragrant taste – and more vitamin C and carotene – and it is easier to tell if they are ripe just by smelling them, or by being naughty and pressing the end of the melon to see if it gives or not.

Pineapples

History has it that Christopher Columbus and his companions were the first Europeans to taste a pineapple when they landed in Guadeloupe. The Indians of the Caribbean had been growing pineapples for ages. They didn't call them pineapples of course. They had a much more sensible name for them. They called them Nana, which means 'flavour'; Nana, Nana , flavour of flavours from which its Latin name, *Ananas comosus* is derived.

Once a food only the wealthy could afford, pineapples are now within the pocket of most of us, at least as a special treat. The best way of choosing a pineapple is to smell it, to make sure that it has the characteristic pineapple aroma. After eating the fruit, it is fun to plant the leaves in a mixture of sand and peat covered with a clear plastic bag as a makeshift propagator to try and grow them on as an ornamental plant.

Whatever their country of origin, all of these fruits are an excellent source of fibre, sugar, minerals and vitamins, including moderate amounts of vitamin C.

Bananas

Along with apples, the fruit we buy most of is the banana. Did you know that 600,000 tons of bananas are eaten in Great Britain every year, and that if you laid all of the bananas grown in the world end to end they would go round the world more than 2,000 times? No? Well, stay with me and you will find lots more useful information like that in this book! With twice as much carbohydrate as most other fruits and nearly 100 kcals, a banana makes an ideal energy rich – but not so energy rich as to be fattening – snack.

Citrus fruits

If it is vitamin C we are after, we should push our trolley along to the citrus fruits – various varieties of orange, grapefruit, lemon and lime are all rich sources.

Lemons were cultivated by the Chinese 3,000 years ago. The lemon and the lime made possible the prevention of scurvy which had been decimating ships' crews at sea on their long voyages of discovery until James Lindt, a Royal Navy surgeon, discovered the remarkable anti-scurvy properties of the fruit. Although most of us landlubbers today will plump for less bitter methods of getting our vitamin C, lemons are still much sought after for creating such culinary delights as lemon meringue pie, and the juice is very useful for keeping sliced apples and bananas looking fresh in the lunch box.

An altogether more palatable citrus fruit with just as much vitamin C as the lemon is the grapefruit. The largest of the citrus fruits, the grapefruit is an essential start to the day for many people. Choose shiny and heavy fruit which give slightly when pressed. They can be stored for a few weeks in a cool place. In the nineteenth century commercial grapefruit plantations were set up in America using seed and plants from the Bahamas and it became a major source of revenue for the states of Arizona, California and Texas. Then, at the beginning of the twentieth century the grapefruit crossed the Atlantic and arrived in Palestine where large orchards were planted. A truly international fruit, the grapefruit in your hand may have hailed from either side of the Atlantic. Even more popular than the grapefruit is the orange which is again rich in vitamin C.

Exotic fruits

Pineapples, bananas and the citrus fruits were all exotic in their day. Fast becoming so familiar in the supermarket as to be in imminent danger of losing their exotic image too are kiwi fruit and mangoes, both of which are excellent sources of vitamin C.

Despite its name, the kiwi fruit originated not in New Zealand but in China. It was not until the beginning of the twentieth century that it arrived in New Zealand where it was extensively planted and rose to become one of the country's major agricultural exports. It was renamed the kiwi fruit by the New Zealanders in 1959, although it is still often known by its earlier and more descriptive name of Chinese gooseberry.

Not so long ago mangoes were a rarity, but they are found in most supermarkets nowadays, and the choice of varieties is increasing. Most people enjoy the texture which is reminiscent of peaches along with the unique taste. As a bonus, at the centre of the fruit is a very interesting seed encased in what looks like a purse, which gives them extra appeal for children.

Custard apple, granadilla, guava, kiwano, kumquat, lychees, mangosteen, pomelo, passion fruit, paw paw, piahaya, physalis, prickly pear, rambutan, sharon fruit, star fruit, ugli fruit. Is there no end to the list of exotic fruits appearing on our supermarket shelves? It's always good to give vent to our inborn spirit of adventure and try new things. A single fruit doesn't cost much so if you find you can't stand the taste it's no great loss, but on the other hand, you might hit the jackpot and discover a new fruit to go on enjoying for years. Go on, gi' 'em a go!

Soft fruit: for sugar, fibre, vitamins and minerals

As we have seen, citrus fruits are a much richer source of vitamin C than home-grown apples and pears so how then did earlier inhabitants of these isles manage to obtain sufficient vitamin C before the development of trade links with other parts of the world? The answer is 'with great difficulty'. Although photographs and video cameras were not around in mediaeval times, artists of the day have provided us with many faithful representations of the features of their subjects which in certain cases show clear evidence of scurvy. In a cold, damp year when fresh fruit and vegetables were in short supply many people suffered it seems from the effects of a lack of vitamin C.

A high vitamin C level is not, however, a characteristic confined to fruits which originate in warm, sunny climates. Strawberries, for instance, have more vitamin C weight for weight than oranges and they grow wild in the Alps. The problem is that in the cool British climate the season for home grown berries is very short and if it is a bad season, producing no surplus for preserving as jam, deficiencies could easily arise during the winter months. Twentieth-century technology ensures that this situation need not arise in Britain today as fresh fruit and vegetables are imported from around the world throughout the year.

Soft fruits like gooseberries, blackberries, raspberries and loganberries (a cross between raspberries and blackberries) are also rich in vitamin C. The richest source of all though is blackcurrants. A pound of blackcurrants contains an unbelievable four times as much vitamin C as a pound of oranges or lemons. Being a bit messy to eat and available only for a relatively short period of the year, cartons of blackcurrant juice tend to be a much more convenient source of vitamin C than the currants themselves nowadays.

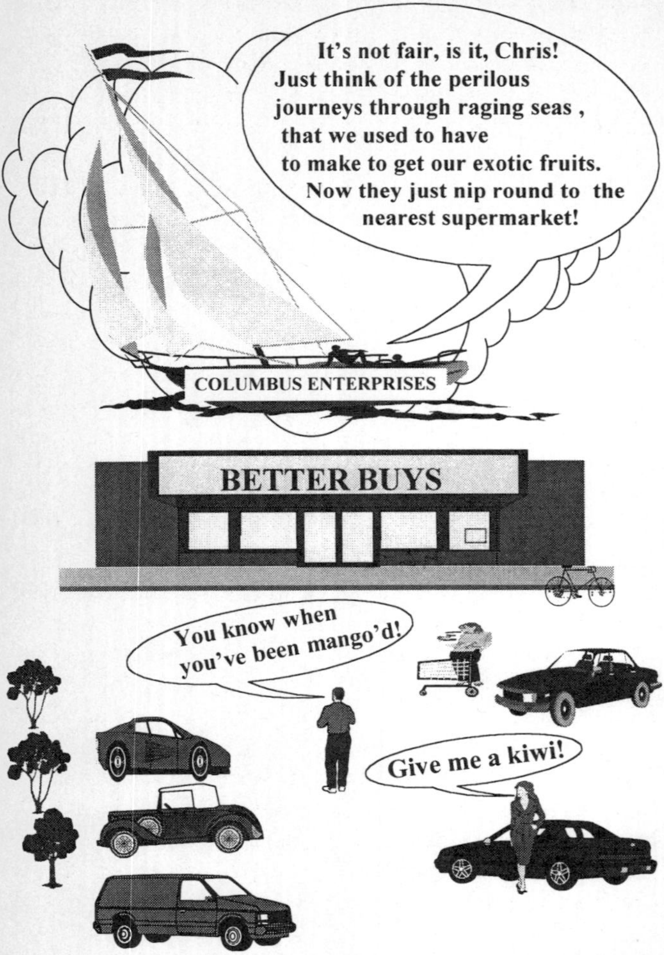
It's not fair, is it, Chris!
Just think of the perilous
journeys through raging seas ,
that we used to have
to make to get our exotic fruits.
Now they just nip round to the
nearest supermarket!
COLUMBUS ENTERPRISES
BETTER BUYS
You know when you've been mango'd!
Give me a kiwi!

As well as being rich in vitamin C, blackberries, raspberries, blackcurrants and other berries are also an excellent source of fibre, with about three times as much as most other fruits. Other types of single berries have also started to appear on the supermarket shelves including blueberry, a great favourite in the United States.

The grape is another soft fruit which has a great deal to offer. As well as vitamins (although they are a bit short on vitamin C), grapes are also a good source of minerals as the vines, being deep rooted, can draw up minerals from deep below the soil long after the top soil has become depleted. Tomatoes are also good.

Most kinds of berries are very rich in vitamin C and fibre but unless we really know for certain that they are safe to eat, the supermarket shelf rather than the hedgerow is the safest place to gather them.

CANNED FRUIT

Canned fruit is almost as good as the real thing; it adds variety and can make a tasty snack. The main problem with it is that it tends to contain added sugar. All is not lost, however, as most manufacturers now offer a choice: the same product bathed, for the sweet-toothed (if they have not all decayed away!) in sugary syrup or, for the weight watcher, in fruit juice. For example, you can buy Del Monte peach halves in sugar and glucose syrup at 72 kcal per 100g or alternatively in juice at 49 kcal. Other brands offer a similar choice. The fact that the peaches are bathed in pineapple juice is neither here nor there. I always go for the healthier option but the choice is yours.

PURE FRUIT JUICE: FOR ENERGY AND VITAMINS, ESPECIALLY VITAMIN C, BUT MAKE SURE IT IS PURE!

Nowadays much, but not all (don't forget the fibre) of the

benefit of fresh fruit can be obtained without actually eating them. The production of pure fruit juice has become a major industry in many countries in recent years and we are now spoiled for choice. No longer limited to the tiny glass bottles of orange and pineapple juice which are now rarely to be found outside the pub, we can buy orange, grapefruit, pineapple, grape, tomato, and mixtures of exotic fruit juices by the litre carton, six at a time, if we want to save money.

Pure fruit juice is an excellent drink. It is a great source of energy for a start. With between 10 and 12 per cent carbohydrate in the form of healthy natural sugar, pure fruit juices are ideal as an energy rich snack, much better than sticky chocolate bars which contain masses of saturated fat as well as the sugar. Did you know that there is as much energy in a litre carton of pure orange juice as in two snack-sized Mars Bars?

There is virtually no fat in pure juice. Like the whole fruit, the pure juice is a rich source of vitamin C, a small glass (150ml) containing half the daily recommended level of the vitamin. Other citrus fruit juices like grapefruit are just as rich in vitamin C as orange juice.

THE UBIQUITOUS WEE CARTONS OF FRUIT JUICE DRINKS – AN INSIPID ALTERNATIVE TO PURE JUICE.

Beware, however, of false imitations. A carton of orange, apple or other drink will only consist of pure juice undiluted by water if it states so directly on the label. It must have the words 'PURE JUICE' or at least 'PURE' somewhere on the carton, otherwise it will almost certainly not be pure juice, so if that is what you want, always make sure that is exactly what it says it is. No other words will do. Don't be deceived by the cartons of similar size with pictures of oranges and blackcurrants which are described as a 'fruit juice drink', 'crush' or just 'orange drink'. The expression 'juice drink' means something completely different.

Most of the juices sold in the one litre cartons are pure juice although there are some prominent exceptions including Ribena fruit juice drinks and tropical juice drinks like Five Alive. Although both of these have water added, they also contain a good helping of fruit juice and are worth drinking.

Unlike the big cartons, most of the drinks sold in small cartons with a straw are fruit juice drinks, not pure juice. There are over a hundred types of these 250ml cartons of fruit juice drinks currently on the market, often suitably festooned with cartoon characters on the box to appeal to children. So if fruit juice drinks do not consist of pure fruit juice, what do they consist of? By law a juice drink need contain no more than 5 per cent fruit juice. The rest can be, and usually is, water and sugar! In practice most brands contain more than the required 5 per cent juice but few have more than 20 per cent. At the moment only about half state on the label how much juice they contain. An exception to the rule tends to be the supermarkets' own brands of orange juice drinks which often contain up to a half fruit juice. One well-known store positions theirs next to the pure juice and craftily call it *Lite* Orange Drink. Of course it's light, half of it is water!

So when you buy a fruit juice drink, what you are getting is in effect a small amount of fruit juice dissolved in water with vitamin C and sugar added to make up for that which would have been provided by the missing fruit. It's a bit like the situation we will encounter later in the guide when we discuss the manufacture of white bread, where the vitamins in the husk are lost when the husk is removed during processing and then added back later. Some fruit juice drink manufacturers go over the top with added vitamins, adding vitamins like B12 and D which weren't there in the first place, and which never occur naturally (unless you include the caterpillars) in fruit and vegetables.

The diet varieties of fruit juice drinks have artificial sweeteners added instead of so much sugar.

I don't want to give the impression that there is anything particularly wrong with the small cartons of juice drinks. Blackcurrant juice for instance is very rich and doesn't have to be taken neat. Ten per cent juice in water gives us quite a lot of juice and compares favourably with the amount of blackcurrants we would be likely to consume if we helped ourselves directly from the bush.

But when it comes to orange juice why pay good money for water and sugar when the pure juice can actually cost less? Most supermarkets sell their own brand of orange juice at a lower price per litre than packs of three 250ml cartons of fruit juice drink. For the school lunch box we can save a pound or two a month by pouring our child pure juice from a litre carton into a plastic flask, rather than giving them disposable 250ml cartons of juice drink, and improve their nutrition to boot. If we have several children we can dilute the pure juice with water to make it even more economical. Pure juice can be diluted with an equal volume of water without losing too much of its taste and without the need to add extra sugar or artificial sweetener. A glass of warm diluted pure orange juice makes a delicious bedtime drink for all the family.

Dentists warn about children eating too many sweets and having too many sweet drinks between meals. Despite this, I would be reluctant to discourage children from enjoying such an eminently healthy snack as pure fruit juice. It is so much better than most of the alternatives like crisps and snack bars which contain too much unhealthy saturated fat. Good dental hygiene is the answer, with regular cleaning.

Always point your trolley in the direction of the *pure* fruit juice, rather than the more insipid fruit juice drinks or bottles of squash for diluting. Most of all, try to avoid loitering around those cans of fizzy, fruit-flavoured drinks, many of which contain no fruit juice at all, just chemical flavourings.

JAMS

Jam is a traditional way of preserving fresh fruit so that its benefits remain available long after it is out of season. As it retains much of the vitamin C of the fresh fruit it probably helped to save thousands of people in the recent past from the misery of scurvy. Today when fresh fruit and vegetables are available in our supermarkets and greengrocers all year round and vitamin C is trapped in cartons of orange juice as well as turning up in all sorts of unlikely places as an additive, jam does not have the same health-giving status. Nevertheless, so long as it is not overdone there is no reason why it should not provide a tasty addition to our diet. The obvious problem with jam is that it has so much sugar, that already present in the fruit being swamped by the huge amount of white sugar added as a preservative. About half of a typical jar of jam is sugar but, as sugar has less than half as many calories as the same weight of fat, and as there is no fat in jam to speak of, the number of calories is less than you might think. One hundred grams of jam provides about 250 kcal, just half what you would get from the same weight of KitKat or Mars Bar.

There are reduced sugar varieties available, but never take a claim of 'reduced sugar' at its face value. Always read the Nutrition Information first. One familiar brand of 'reduced sugar strawberry jam' has slightly more sugar than, for instance, 'Robinson's strawberry jam' which makes no such claim. Lower sugar options are to be had, like Tesco's which has one third sugar instead of the typical one half. Diabetic jams are also available with virtually no sugar, the sugar being replaced by an equal weight of the bulk sweetener sorbitol which is used in many diabetic foods. But for those who do not have diabetes it is unlikely that they offer any real advantage.

To find out how much vitamin C there is in fresh fruit, nip along to Chapter 4, *The Vitamin and Mineral Jungle.*

CHAPTER 3

The Vegetable Section

Official Recommendation: We should (as a population) double the amount of fresh and frozen vegetables we eat.

In the Department of Health's Health Survey, two out of three people reported eating vegetables every day, so we obviously do a lot better with vegetables than we do with fruit. Even so, one in ten people said they eat vegetables less than three times a week. We still have a long way to go, therefore, to achieve the recommendation that: *the combined number of helpings of fruit and vegetables should be at least five a day*. Five a day is the healthy way, so let's go for five and stay alive!

POTATOES: RICH IN STARCH, PROTEIN AND VITAMIN C

No supermarket vegetable section would be complete without a ton or so of what was for long the staple diet of millions of people in Britain. Yes, you've got it, the potato. Introduced from South America in the sixteenth century, it eventually became the main source of carbohydrate and protein for large sections of the British population. Then disaster struck in the shape of potato blight which year after year obliterated much of the crop. Thousands starved while others migrated to America. This tragedy illustrates the importance of not relying too heavily on just one or two sources of food, as excellent as they might be.

Many different varieties of potatoes are grown on our farms. Varieties which are high in starch and low in sugar are preferred for crisp and chip making, while canners require small varieties of potatoes which are low in starch with a waxy flesh to withstand the canning process. Other varieties are chosen for their resistance to drought or disease.

Unlike wheat and most other cereal crops, only about a quarter of the potatoes grown on British farms are in fact processed, the bulk of the crop being sold directly to us as natural raw potato and that is just how it should be. Potatoes, like other root vegetables and cereals, are an excellent source of the starch we should be obtaining most of our energy from.

Now for something which not everyone realises. Potatoes are also an excellent source of vitamin C. New potatoes straight from the soil have half as much, weight for weight, as some citrus fruits. The vitamin content falls with storage and still more can be lost on boiling, but even so, as we as a nation tend to eat a lot of potatoes, they are an important, inexpensive, natural source of vitamin C for millions of people in this country.

The bad news is that the consumption of raw potatoes has been falling relentlessly. We now buy only about two thirds as many as we did twenty years ago, despite the fact that most of us now have cars to carry them home in. Boiled or baked, potatoes are an inexpensive, highly nutritious part of our diet, so if you are one of those responsible for the falling consumption, think again!

CHIPS

What about chips? Chips are a nutritionist's nightmare, a classic example, like crisps, of how to convert the superbly healthy potato into something far less desirable. Having said that, many of the brands of frozen oven-ready chips now threatening, cuckoo fashion, to displace everything else from the supermarket freezers contain less than 5 per cent fat overall and less than 1 per cent of the undesirable, saturated kind, so eaten in moderation they are not really that bad. They are certainly a great improvement on the chips so often served up in chippies and restaurants and those typically prepared at home which are usually plastered with saturated fat and should be approached with caution.

CARROTS, PARSNIPS, TURNIPS AND OTHER ROOT VEGETABLES

All of the root crops in the vegetable section – not just potatoes – are an inexpensive source of the starch that the World Health Organisation says we should be obtaining most of our energy from. Turnips, swedes, beetroot, carrots and parsnips are good, nutritious foods packed with energy-yielding starch, fibre, protein and vitamins.

It is a pity that the raw turnips on sale usually have the size and texture of ten-pin bowling balls, when there are dozens of small, tasty, bite-size varieties available. But with the recent introduction to the vegetable section of miniature varieties of vegetables like sweetcorn, cabbages and carrots, mini turnips will no doubt soon follow and we shall be able to return the vice, hacksaw, hammer and chisel to their rightful place in the tool shed. Joking apart, once chopped up into small chunks and boiled, the bowling ball turnips become soft and tasty and well worth the effort.

Happily, parsnips and carrots are no trouble at all to prepare. If not organically grown, we just need to peel and top and tail them to get rid of any pesticide residues and there we are. We should eat more of them along with our potatoes.

Carrots are a particularly interesting vegetable as they

are a major source of a substance called beta-carotene which our bodies can convert into vitamin A. It is this beta-carotene which gives carrots their red colour. As well as being an antioxidant (more about antioxidants later), vitamin A is essential for the proper functioning of the eyes. In many parts of the world, vitamin A deficiency is a major cause of blindness, a needless tragedy as it can so easily be prevented, even where the diet is poor, by supplements of the vitamin. I will spare you the old joke about rabbits never being seen wearing glasses!

Beta-carotene is absorbed from our intestines better in the presence of fat, so it is a nice idea to make a habit of adding some grated carrot to any dish we prepare using vegetable oil or to a dish which will be followed by small amounts of a fatty dessert like ice cream. Carrots do not of course have to be cooked. There are lots of very tasty varieties which we can eat raw, either grated as suggested above or, if we like a good crunch, just as they are.

The good news is that although the consumption of potatoes has fallen, that of other fresh vegetables has remained steady.

EAT YOUR GREENS

Now for the greens. I hope you always eat your greens. Greens are a very good source of roughage and vitamins, including beta-carotene, vitamin C and the folic acid which, as we shall see in the next chapter, is so essential during pregnancy. It's worth remembering that the amount of vitamin we obtain depends not only on how much the vegetable contains in every 100 grams, but how much is lost in cooking before we eat it and how much of it we actually eat. Parsley is very rich in vitamin C, but because we tend to eat so little of it, it is not likely to be a significant source of the vitamin. Potatoes, on the other hand, have only about a tenth as much vitamin C as the same weight of parsley, but because we eat hundreds of times as much they provide us with a substantial amount of the vitamin.

My favourite green leafy vegetable is lettuce. I love brown lettuce sandwiches. It's the bread that's brown, not the lettuce, of course! The great advantage of lettuce over most leafy vegetables is that it is usually eaten raw without any of the beta-carotene (which we can convert into vitamin A) and vitamin C being lost as a result of cooking.

Chinese cabbages, which can be eaten as a salad vegetable like lettuces, are now available in most supermarkets. In case you have any qualms about Chinese methods of fertilising the soil – Sh... you know what! – Chinese refers to the variety rather than the immediate country of origin. British cabbages, both red and green, can be eaten raw too. They can be grated and added to salads along with grated carrots, apples and so on, but for some reason they usually end up boiled. A pound of raw cabbage contains as much vitamin C as a pound of oranges. Better still, Brussels sprouts have twice as much! To avoid losing most of the precious vitamin C, it is important to remember to boil for as short a time and in as little water as possible, and why not go one step further and re-use the water for making soup or just drink it neat rather than pour its vitamins and minerals down the sink.

The ancestors of the supermarket lettuces and cabbages still grow wild, but the wild varieties are nowhere near as huge and football-like as the iceberg lettuces and cabbages of the supermarket. These crops are the result of years of selective breeding to produce as much green leaf on as small an area of land as possible, a strategy which has obviously proven very successful and provided us with the not-to-be-missed opportunity of making a substantial helping of green leaves a regular part of our diet.

Cauliflowers and broccoli are also a good buy. Pound for pound they too, when fresh, have as much vitamin C as oranges. A boiled cauliflower and grated, half-fat cheese makes an excellent light meal. Not too much cheese though and go gently with the boiling.

Spinach is another leafy vegetable that is readily obtainable, and has the reputation for being a good source of iron. All greens have a fair amount, but spinach has about three times as much iron as most other vegetables. Unfortunately, the iron in spinach is in a form which it is difficult for us to absorb from our intestines. Spinach is also very rich in beta-carotene for making vitamin A, being pound for pound one of the richest sources after carrots. Curly kale and red peppers also have exceptionally large amounts of beta-carotene.

RAW VEGETABLES

The benefits of raw vegetables cannot be stressed too strongly, simply because eating them raw avoids the loss of vitamins and minerals in cooking. A good way of allowing children to eat them is to provide a dish full of sliced or grated carrot, apple, pepper, cucumber, lettuce, cabbage, water cress, celery, tomato, whatever is available, on the dinner table to tuck into while they are waiting for the main meal. That will ensure a good daily intake of beta-carotene, vitamin C and other vitamins and minerals.

FINGER ON THE PULSE — PEAS AND BEANS

Most supermarkets have a very limited selection of fresh pulses – the collective term for peas and beans – but this deficiency is more than compensated for by the abundance of dried and frozen pulses.

Whether fresh, dried, frozen, canned or processed,

peas and beans are something we should be eating more of. The reason for this is that when the protein in pulses is mixed with cereal protein the result is a top-quality protein which is better than either eaten alone.

Pulse protein plus cereal protein: the perfect combination

Proteins, as you may be aware, are made up of 20 different kinds of amino acids linked together side by side in a chain. Imagine a necklace made up of 20 different kinds of beads folded up in the palm of your hand and you will have some idea of what a protein looks like. Different proteins differ in the number of each kind of amino acids (the beads) they contain and the order in which they are arranged along the chain.

The protein in red meat, fish, poultry, milk and milk products and egg whites contains all of the amino acids we need to make the protein in our own bodies, for building muscles and making enzymes etc. Nutritionists refer to it as 'first class protein'. The protein in cereal grains, however, tends to be low in one of the amino acids called lysine, so we would not be able to stay healthy indefinitely on cereals if we were to eat nothing else besides. Similarly, the protein in peas and beans contains very little of an amino acid called methionine so again we could not stay healthy if we were to eat nothing but peas and beans.

Mix and match

The good news, however, is that cereal proteins contain the methionine lacking in pulses, and pulse proteins contain the lysine lacking in cereals, so by simply mixing the two together we can obtain all of the amino acids we need. If you look at the label on a typical loaf of supermarket bread you will find that it is made from wheat flour that has been supplemented with soya bean flour in recognition of this fact.

Cereals and pulses should ideally be eaten at the same meal, but if we can't manage that, we can have cereals for breakfast, balanced with peas and beans or other vegetables for dinner. Alternatively, just adding semi-skimmed milk to our cereal will have a similar effect, with the lysine in the milk proteins making up for the lack of it in the cereals.

Vegetarians have long known that the secret of staying healthy on a vegetarian diet is to eat as wide a range of food as possible, which is equally good advice whatever our eating pattern.

Bean sprouts

Getting back to the beans though, I like all kinds but my favourite are bean sprouts.

The Chinese are very fond of their bean sprouts as you will know if you have ever eaten in a Chinese restaurant, and with good reason. They are rich in vitamins and easily digested protein and, what is more, are absolutely delicious and very cheap to prepare.

Preparing bean sprouts is simplicity itself. The first thing, obviously, is to buy the mung or adjuki beans from a supermarket or wholefood store.

When you get them back home, take a couple of handfuls of the beans, wash them in cold water, then soak overnight in tepid water. Next morning, rinse again and drain off any excess water. Place several layers of paper towelling (the unbleached kind made with recycled paper is ideal) over the bottom of a shallow tray, dampen the paper thoroughly, pour off excess water, and sprinkle the beans over the surface. Cover the tray with a plastic bag and place it in a completely dark, warm spot such as an airing cupboard. Inspect occasionally to make sure that the paper remains damp and that there is not any free water at the base of the tray. After about three days, remove the tray and place it in a brightly lit spot for a day or two until the sprouts turn green. Give them a rinse and they are ready to eat, either on their own, or mixed with other vegetable or in salads.

It is not only beans that can be sprouted. Alfalfa is another favourite which has the flavour of fresh garden peas. Then there is fenugreek, radish and the familiar mustard and cress. These last five can be sprouted in the dark at room temperature without extra heat. See what is available in your supermarket or health food store, but don't experiment. Eat only the sprouts of seeds that are sold specifically for sprouting as others may be poisonous.

FROZEN VEGETABLES

To supplement the fresh vegetables, most supermarkets also have a long convoy of freezers loaded with packets of frozen vegetables, which have an embarrassing habit of tearing and releasing their contents when you pick them up to read the label.

It is significant that the authors of the government reports, in recommending that as a nation we should greatly increase the amount of vegetables we eat, did not differentiate between fresh and frozen vegetables. That was deliberate. The reason is that frozen vegetables are as good nutritionally as fresh, because freezing vegetables when they are still fresh traps the vitamins and prevents the levels falling significantly until they are thawed out and cooked.

Salt is sometimes added to the vegetables, so always check the packets for the low salt brands.

Frozen vegetables are one convenience food that I can heartily recommend. There is a tremendous variety to choose from, and we can obtain an interesting mixture such as peas, beans, and sweetcorn all in a single packet. They are so convenient, no preparation necessary. Just snip open the packet, pop the vegetables into a pan of boiling water and a few minutes later, there are the peas, beans, Brussels sprouts – you name it – ready to eat.

Many people are put off eating fresh peas, beans and Brussels sprouts because of the time and effort involved in their preparation. This a pity because, despite being so fiddly to prepare, they are amongst the most nutritious of foods. Peas and beans are second only to whole grain cereals in fibre content to keep our bowels moving, and as we have seen, eaten along with cereals, they provide first-class protein. It is good to see that with frozen vegetables all of the hard work has been done for us.

The value of frozen vegetables needs to be more widely recognised. They contain the same vitamins and minerals as fresh vegetables, are inexpensive, and so incredibly easy to prepare that there is absolutely no excuse for not eating more of them.

CANNED VEGETABLES

Even canned vegetables are not to be scoffed at, so long as there aren't too many additives like salt and sugar, so always check the label. Many manufacturers now provide the option of buying their product with less salt and less sugar than the standard product. The two options are usually to be found side by side on the shelves, often at exactly the same price. Let us look at some cans of baked beans and see how they differ. The table below compares three brands of baked beans which I found in a local supermarket each of which was available both with the usual high levels of salt and sugar and as a healthier option with lower salt and sugar.

Brand	**Salt g/100g**	**Sugar g/100g**	**Artificial sweetener**	**Calories kcal/100g**
Tesco in tomato sauce	0.5	6.0	None	96
Tesco low sugar, low salt	0.3	3.5	Saccharin	84
HP ordinary in tomato sauce	0.48	6.1	None	85
HP Healthy	0.34	1.7	Acesulfame K	65
Heinz with tomato sauce	0.5	6.0	None	75
Heinz Weight Watchers	0.3	0.7	Saccharin	56

As regards salt there is nothing to choose between brands. In all three healthy options the amount of salt has been reduced by nearly a half. The healthy options also have less added sugar, but exactly how much less varies enormously between brands. Heinz Weight Watchers beans contains only one fifth as much sugar as the Tesco low sugar variety and only about two thirds as many calories, so it lives up to its name. It is generally agreed that most of us consume too much salt, so definitely go for the low salt options. Whether you want to go further and choose the brands with the lowest amount of sugar depends on the extent of your aversion to added sugar and how keenly you are watching the calories. If you want to avoid both added sugar and artificial sweeteners, tough luck! As they take away the sugar with one hand, manufacturers insist on adding artificial sweeteners with the other.

If you are keen, you could produce a little table like the one above for all of the products you buy regularly. Focus on one product a week, record the vital statistics of the different brands on offer at your local supermarket in a notebook and select which is best for you. Then the next time you go shopping you can just make a beeline for the favoured brand.

If you want to do the same thing in the comfort of your own home, you can do as I did and buy all six cans, or however many varieties there are of the product you are looking at, just the once, and compare the taste as well. If it sounds like a lot of work, divide the task up amongst your friends. Form a Healthy Option Club which meets for coffee (or preferably pure orange juice) once a week for a chat and to exchange notes!

Award a prize for the most confusing label. What about this for starters: 'Sweetcorn in Sugared Salt Water' and the Healthy Eating variety 'Sweetcorn in Water, No Added Sugar or Salt'. Sure enough the healthy option contains no salt compared with 0.3 g per 100g in the other but, according to the nutrition information table, the amount of sugar is exactly the same in both! How can a sugared product contain the same amount of sugar as one with no added sugar? Work that one out!

A few days after I spotted this, a headline in *The Scotsman* ran 'Food labelling laws have cost (name of supermarket) deer'. It had been found that venison reared and slaughtered in New Zealand was being shipped to Britain to be packaged and labelled by the supermarket as: 'Produce of the UK'. Their venison had previously been reared in the UK, but when their suppliers had started importing from New Zealand they had forgotten to change the label! With thousands of products on the shelves, errors are bound to creep in from time to time, so it's important not to accept things at their face value and always to query with the manufacturers labels which don't seem to us to be quite right. They usually appreciate these things being politely pointed out, particularly if it gives them the opportunity to rectify the situation before the press get hold of it.

As a general rule, fresh vegetables taste the best, but frozen vegetables are as good nutritionally, and dried and canned worth keeping as a back-up for times when you can't get out to the supermarket to buy fresh or frozen.

GARDEN VEGETABLES VERSUS SUPERMARKET VEGETABLES

The question is often asked whether supermarket vegetables are as good as those you grow in your own garden.

Let there be no mistake, supermarket vegetables are excellent and we should be eating more of them, but the vegetables we grow in our own garden, if we are lucky enough to have a garden, can be even better.

There are two main nutritional advantages of garden-grown vegetables, both relating to vitamin levels.The first is that they can be picked while they are young and tender, when vitamin levels tend to be at their highest, whereas by the time they are harvested commercially the levels will have fallen somewhat.

The second advantage is that vegetables from the garden can be eaten within minutes of picking so you can be sure that virtually none of the vitamin has been lost. Supermarket vegetables and greens have much the same amount of protein and carbohydrate as they had when first harvested, but vitamin levels start falling slowly after harvesting, so the sooner we can get our teeth into them the better. Frozen vegetables, however, keep their original vitamin levels longer.

But we eat for pleasure as well as nutrition, so another reason for growing a few vegetables of our own is that they often taste better. Why is that? Apart from being able to pick them when they are young and tender, one of the main reasons is that they contain sugar which, after they are picked, changes into starch. This is especially noticeable with sweetcorn which really is as sweet as its name suggests when first picked and eaten straightaway, but within minutes, the taste starts to suffer as the sugar is converted into starch.

It takes a lot to beat the taste of a fresh young carrot, still warm from the soil. Get a good seed catalogue like the well-known Thompson and Morgans, for advice on which vegetable varieties taste the best raw. Most root vegetables, including potatoes, taste good raw if harvested while they are still young and tender but most of the more mature supermarket root vegetables need cooking to make them more palatable.

Another explanation for the better taste is that when we are cultivating vegetables in our own garden or allotment, we are free to choose which varieties to grow. We can if we wish go for the variety with the best taste even though it might not have the highest yield. Farmers, on the other hand need to make a profit, so will almost always opt for the higher yielding variety or the one most resistant to pests even if its taste is not quite so good as the alternatives.

Don't let me put you off supermarket vegetables though. Despite their generally poorer taste and slightly lower vitamin levels, they are still nutritionally one of the best foods around, packed with carbohydrate and protein, fibre, vitamins and minerals. Remember the official advice is that nationally our consumption of fresh and frozen vegetables, whether they come from the supermarket, the local greengrocers or our own gardens, should double.

CHAPTER 4

The Vitamin and Mineral Jungle

DO WE NEED EXTRA VITAMINS?

What's this? A shelf full of bottles of vitamin pills in a supermarket brimming over with fresh food. Shouldn't a good, varied diet already contain all of the vitamins we need? Indeed it should, but there is probably no harm in taking extra vitamin pills occasionally or a vitamin-rich extract like cod liver oil with its vitamins A, D and E, just to make sure, so long as we don't overdo them. If we are vegetarians our intake of vitamin D and vitamin B12 could be on the low side, so a supplement of these may be worth considering. If we do take extra vitamins we should take care never to exceed the amount recommended by the manufacturers on the bottle.

In our expedition to the fruit and vegetable sections we were keen to extol the virtues of foods rich in vitamin C and beta-carotene (which our bodies convert into vitamin A), but let us now run through the other major vitamins as well and remind ourselves why we need them and what foods they are to be found in.

It is a good memory aid to organise the vitamins into groups.

In Search of Vitamins

Vitamin

A Beta-carotene from carrots and green leafy veg. Vitamin A from animal products.

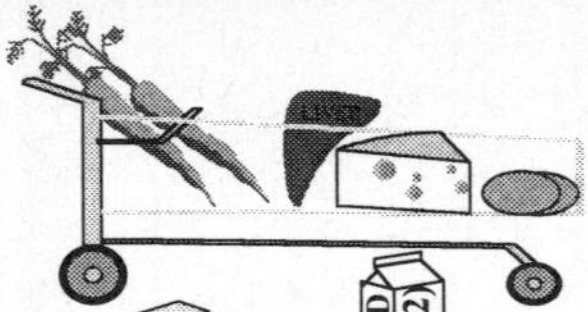

B Most foods, especially whole cereal products and yeast.

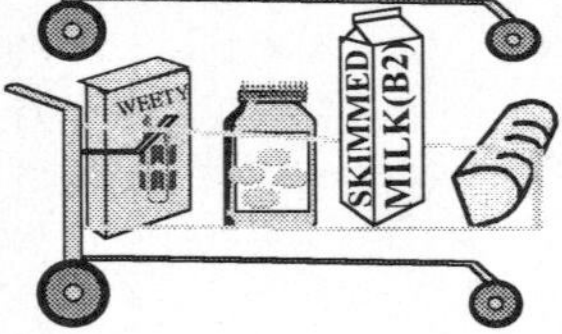

B12 Animal products and fortified cereals.

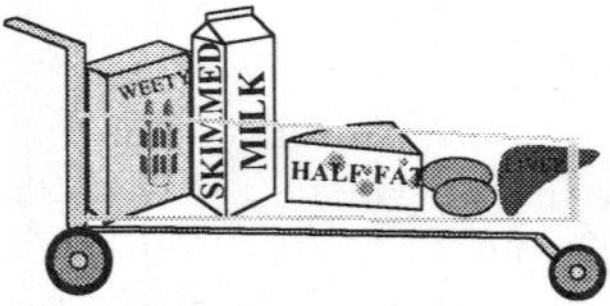

C Fresh and frozen fruit and veg and pure fruit juices.

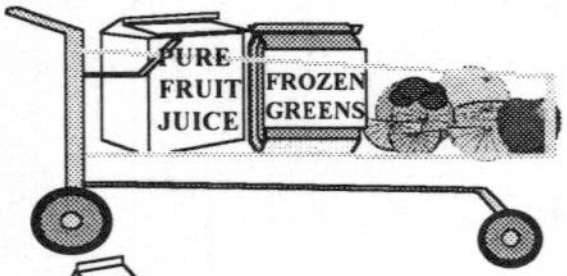

D Sunshine, eggs, dairy products and oily fish.

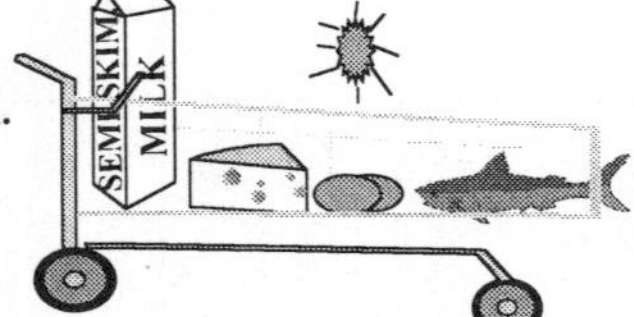

P

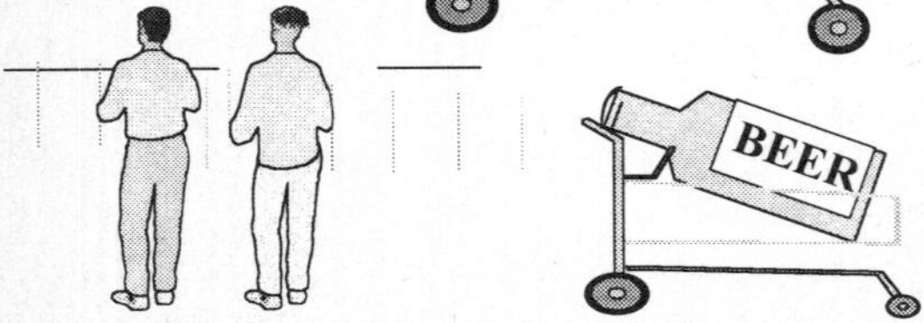

RECOMMENDED DAILY AMOUNTS

Before we go any further, a note on what the expression 'Recommended daily amount' at the bottom of each table means. The exact amount of a particular vitamin, mineral or other nutrient that is needed varies from one person to another. It depends on such factors as our age, sex, build, level of activity, the climate, as well as individual differences in our biochemistry. It also depends on what other food we eat, as some substances in the diet interfere with the absorption of certain vitamins and minerals from the intestines into the bloodstream and, as we shall see, vitamins and minerals can even interfere with each other's absorption. It is, therefore, impossible to state exactly how much of a vitamin etc. we need each day.

Despite the difficulty, a number of nutritional and government organisations, based on the available evidence, have set what are known as Recommended Daily Amounts (sometimes now referred to as 'Reference Nutrient Intakes'). At the end of each of the tables in this chapter I have included for each vitamin the Recommended Daily Amount agreed by the European Community. Unfortunately, there is no worldwide agreement and for some nutrients, notably vitamin C, the USA recommendations are higher than the European.

Now, beware of falling into the trap of thinking that the Recommended Daily Amount is the amount you must eat every day to stay healthy. In setting Recommended Daily Amounts the experts err on the side of safety and set them at a level which will be sufficient for almost everybody, even those with much higher than average needs. Most of us, therefore, will be able to stay healthy on somewhat less than the Recommended Daily Amount. Although they are imprecise, these figures nevertheless provide a useful guide as to the sort of amount of a particular nutrient we should be aiming at.

VITAMINS A, C AND E — THE ACE VITAMINS

Our first group consists of vitamins A, C and E. This spells ACE so we can call them the ACE vitamins. It is a silly but convenient way of remembering that these three vitamins have something important in common. They all act as antioxidants, substances which interact in the body with damaging forms of chemicals known as free radicals rendering them harmless. Evidence is accumulating that the ACE vitamins may help to protect against the sort of damage to living cells which may eventually lead to certain forms of cancer and heart disease. You may have noticed this word 'antioxidant' on the labels of processed foods, especially those which contain fats, like powdered milk. The purpose of antioxidants in such foods is to prevent them from going off. The antioxidant used is often vitamin C, usually referred to when occupying this role by its formal scientific name of L-ascorbic acid.

Vitamin A

As well as being an antioxidant, vitamin A, as we revealed in our discussion of the virtues of carrots, has another important role. In many poorer parts of the world a severe lack of the vitamin in the diet is one of the main causes of blindness.

Ready-made vitamin A is found in fish oils and dairy produce but, as can be seen from the table following, by far the biggest source is liver. Just a mouthful of liver will keep us going for weeks. This includes chicken liver. That little bag of giblets which always used to come with the chicken was an excellent source of vitamin A, not to mention vitamin B12 and iron, but unfortunately it has been outlawed by the European Community on the grounds of hygiene.

If you take supplements of vitamin A, never exceed the stated dose as it is toxic in large amounts. This was discovered to their cost by the early Arctic explorers. They knew that the native Eskimos never ate the liver of the polar bears they hunted but thought they were just being silly, so they went ahead and tucked into it. As a result, they became violently ill, the reason being that polar bear liver contains enormous amounts of vitamin A on account, no doubt, of all of the oily fish they eat. So when you are next in your local supermarket be sure to steer clear of the polar bear liver! The more familiar kinds of liver are good for us in moderation most of the time, but owing to its high vitamin A content, the current advice is that liver should be avoided during pregnancy or at least eaten then in only very small amounts.

If you are a vegetarian, there is no need to worry about vitamin A as it is not absolutely essential to consume the ready-made vitamin. We are all DIY experts capable of making it ourselves with our biochemical tool kit from the beta-carotene found in all dark green leafy vegetables and in root vegetables, especially carrots. Peppers are also a very rich source.

The various forms of the vitamin occur in such a wide variety of products that there is hardly any need to go actively searching for it. It will find us! So long as we eat lots of fresh vegetables along with just a little fat or oil to aid the absorption of the beta-carotene from our intestines we should not go short.

WHERE TO AIM YOUR TROLLEY TO FIND READY MADE VITAMIN A IN THE SUPERMARKET

	Micrograms of vitamin A in each 100 gm (3.5oz) of food
Liver and liver products	
Liver, calf	30,000
Lamb, ox and pig liver	16,000 to 20,000
Chicken liver	11,000
Liver paté	7,300
Liver sausage	2,600
Haggis	1,800
Faggots	460
Cod liver oil	18,000 (about 900 in a 5ml teaspoon)
Eggs and egg products	
Whole, raw chicken eggs	190 (about 2 grade 6 eggs) All in the yolk
Whole, raw duck eggs	540
Omelette and quiche	Around 200
Gateau	Around 250
Milk and dairy products	
Full fat milk*	52 (about 300 in a pint)
Semi-skimmed milk	21 (about 120 in a pint)
Skimmed milk	1 (hardly any)
Butter*	815
Margarine	780
Low fat spread	920
Double cream*	600
Cheese, Cheddar (half fat)	160
Dairy vanilla ice cream	115

**Avoid, as these contain too much saturated fat*

RECOMMENDED DAILY AMOUNT: 800 MICROGRAMS
(OR DIY FROM BETA-CAROTENE)

VITAMIN C

Like vitamin A, vitamin C also has an important role as an antioxidant mopping up free radicals, and there is considerable medical interest in whether it can help to protect against certain kinds of cancer. Clinical trials are currently under way to determine whether large doses of the vitamin can help to prevent what are known as pre-cancerous lesions, that is changes in the body with an increased risk of developing into cancer, from actually doing so, but it is too early to say yet whether there is anything in the idea.

In our voyage of discovery through the fruit section, we remarked about James Lindt's recognition of the anti-scurvy properties of lemons and limes. It was not until the early nineteen thirties, a century and a half later, that the fruits' remarkable properties could be attributed to their high vitamin C content. It was not only adventurous seafarers deprived of fresh fruit and vegetables who suffered from scurvy in times past, but ordinary townsfolk too. Mediaeval portraits often depict the skin sores characteristic of the disease. People living in Northern areas would have been especially susceptible after a cold, damp spell when fresh fruit supplies were limited. Nowadays, few people in Britain consume so little vitamin C that they come down with the severest forms of scurvy common in mediaeval times but some, typically as a result of self-neglect due, for instance, to chronic alcoholism still manage to consume such small amounts as to render themselves susceptible to internal bruising, poor healing of wounds and bleeding gums. Many people believe from personal experience that vitamin C helps to prevent them from catching colds, but it has proven surprisingly difficult to prove this scientifically.

The problem with vitamin C is that we need a regular

daily supply as, unlike vitamin A, we are not able to store it in our bodies. This is no problem to those of us who eat fresh fruit and vegetables daily and drink pure fruit juices, but people on a junk food diet can easily go short.

It is puzzling, however, how some people seem to consume hardly any of the fresh foods which contain vitamin C yet show no signs of deficiency. This is probably because large amounts of the vitamin (usually described as L-ascorbic acid on the label) are added to some processed foods such as bread, tinned fruit, fizzy drinks, powdered potatoes and powdered milk either as an antioxidant to prevent fats going off or to replace the naturally occurring vitamin which has been lost in processing.

The daily intake recommended in the European Community is 60 mg per day. Taking more than this does not appear to have any harmful effects as the excess is just excreted.

As we navigated our way through the international waters of the fruit and vegetable section I pointed out many of the richest sources of vitamin C. These are summarised in the table below. We should expect to lose about a third of the vitamin C when the vegetables are gently boiled. Greens and other vegetables will also gradually lose their vitamin C if kept in a warm room, so they should always be kept in the fridge until ready to eat.

WHERE TO AIM YOUR TROLLEY TO FIND VITAMIN C IN THE SUPERMARKET

	Milligrams of vitamin C in each 100gm (3.5 oz) of food
The Vegetable Section	
Red peppers	140
Green peppers	120
Brussels sprouts, fresh	115
frozen	115
Curly kale	110
Broccoli	87
Cabbage	49
Cauliflower	43
Mange tout peas	54
Other peas	24
Parsnips	17
New potatoes	16 (modest levels but we eat a lot,
Old potatoes	11 freshly dug contain about 21mg)
Tomatoes	17
Parsley	190 (high levels but we tend to eat very small amounts)
Watercress	62
Most other vegetables	10-30
The Fruit Section	
Blackcurrants	200
Strawberries	77
Lemons	58
Oranges, Clementines	54
Lychees	45
Grapefruit	36
Canteloupe melon	26
Raspberries	32
Apples	2 to 20 depending on variety
Most other fruit	10 to 20

Fruit Juices	
Pure orange juice,	20
Ribena blackcurrant fruit juice drink	30 A small glass (200ml) provides the EC, RDA
Five Alive fruit juice drink	8
Most squashes and other non-pure fruit juices are fortified with vitamin C	
Less obvious sources	
Processed fruit and vegetables	
Jam	10
Frozen chips	16
Instant powdered potatoes	23 fortified
Crisps	27
Added to a few breakfast cereals	*(not normally present in cereals)*
Bran flakes	50
Weetos	30
Fortified milk	*(not normally much present in milk)*
Fortified UHT milk	35
Dried skimmed milk	13
Bread	Used as an improving agent in flour
Fruit pies and canned fruit	Wide variation in amounts

RECOMMENDED DAILY AMOUNT IN ADULTS: 60 MILLIGRAMS

Vitamin E

In common with the other ACE vitamins, vitamin E is an antioxidant assisting our bodies in their fight against free radicals and thereby possibly helping to protect against a whole range of diseases, including cancer, and heart disease. We have the makings of a new exciting computer game here!

People who eat a lot of polyunsaturated fat have an increased need for vitamin E but, fortunately, foods like vegetable oils which are high in polyunsaturates also tend to be naturally high in vitamin E.

Where do we look for vitamin E? Virtually all food whether it is obtained from animals or plants contains a significant amount of vitamin E so it is just about impossible to suffer from a severe deficiency of it on anything other than a starvation diet. The few foods which hardly contain any are white bread and white rice and sweets.The table below gives an idea of where to aim your trolley for the richest sources.

WHERE TO AIM YOUR TROLLEY TO FIND VITAMIN E IN THE SUPERMARKET

	Milligrams of vitamin E in each 100gm (3.5 oz) of food
Cod Liver Oil: (Seven Seas)	100 (5 in a 5ml teaspoon)

DON'T EAT COOKING OILS AND MARGARINE SPECIALLY TO GET VITAMIN E AS THEY INCREASE THE NEED FOR IT, SO IT TENDS TO BE SELF-DEFEATING.

Cooking Oils	
Wheatgerm oil	137
Sunflower seed oil	49
Cotton seed and Safflower oil	42
Soya, Corn, Peanut and Rapeseed oil	16 to 22
Margarine	8
Eggs	1 (about 0.5 in a grade 6 egg)
Nuts and Seeds (without shells)	
Sunflower seeds	38
Hazelnuts	25
Almonds	24

Peanuts	10
Brazil nuts	7
Marzipan	6
The Fruit and Vegetable Section	
Sweet potato	5
Blackberries	2
Spinach	2
Mangoes	1
Pears	0.5
High Fibre Breakfast Cereals	
All-Bran	2
Muesli Swiss style	3
Salad Dressings	
Mayonnaise	19 (about 20 teaspoons)
Salad cream	10 (about 20 teaspoons)

RECOMMENDED DAILY AMOUNT 10 MILLIGRAMS

VITAMIN D — THE SUNSHINE VITAMIN

The second group of vitamins has only one member, vitamin D, the sunshine vitamin, which is present in full fat milk and semi-skimmed milk (but not skimmed milk) and in milk products like half fat cheese, as well as in fish. DIY enthusiasts will be heartened to learn that we can also make it ourselves in our skin with the help of ultraviolet light.

As we learned from our school history books, in the early days of industrialisation, children in London and Glasgow and other big cities often suffered from rickets, a disease characterised by failure of the bones to develop properly. The cause of this was a deficiency of vitamin D and calcium which arose because they were not able to obtain a balanced diet containing enough of the fish and milk products which contain these nutrients. The lack of vitamin D would not have mattered if they had been exposed to adequate sunshine to allow them to make it in their skin, but they lived in tall tenements which shielded them from what little sunlight managed to penetrate the air pollution emanating from the factories and coal fires, and holidays in Benidorm or Tenerife were unheard of.

So despite recent killjoy skin cancer prevention campaigns, sunshine is not all bad but, like everything else, it needs to be taken in moderation.

Vitamin D deficiency can sometimes be a problem even today for people with dark skin living in Britain because it takes more sunshine to produce the vitamin in dark skin than it does in white. If for religious reasons or because they cannot tolerate milk sugar or proteins, they are unable to eat dairy products, the risk is greater. Vitamin D deficiency can also arise in people who are housebound and unable to get out in the sunshine. If you do the shopping for an elderly relative or neighbour, if possible, go for the brands with vitamin D supplements.

For people at risk of vitamin D deficiency there is, however, a good old-fashioned remedy — cod liver oil.

Don't groan too loud. We can always mix it up in a yoghurt or a glass of orange juice if we don't like the taste, or buy pots of malt extract and cod liver oil, which most people find much tastier than the neat oil. Yes, it's good stuff, cod liver oil, packed not only with vitamins A, D and E but also with the omega-3 essential fatty acids. More about the omega-3 essential fatty acids later. Cod liver oil will not be necessary if we are including plenty of salmon, trout, mackerel, sardines, tuna and other oily fish, either fresh or in cans, in our diet, or being blessed with more summers like that of 1995 which enable us to get out and about in the sunshine.

WHERE TO FIND VITAMIN D IN THE SUPERMARKET ON A RAINY DAY. ON A SUNNY DAY, JUST RELAX IN THE GARDEN AND MAKE YOUR OWN!

	Micrograms of vitamin D in each 100gm (3.5oz) of food
Cod Liver Oil	210 (10 in a 5ml teaspoon)
The Fish Counter	
Oily fish–herring, kipper and mackerel	Between 15 and 25
Canned salmon	13
Canned pilchards and sardines	8
White fish	Just a trace
Margarine: artificially fortified	8
Eggs	
Ducks	5
Hens	2
Breakfast Cereals : fortified	Read the labels
Eg Kelloggs Corn Flakes, Coco Pops & Rice Crispies	2.8
Beverages: fortified	
Complan, Horlicks and Ovaltine	2 per 100 gm powder About 0.25 made up
Milk and Dairy Products	
Butter	0.8
Cheese	0.2
Vanilla ice cream	0.1
Full fat goats' milk	0.1
Full fat cows' milk	0.03
Semi-skimmed cows milk	0.01
Enriched semi-skimmed milk. eg Marks and Spencer	0.03
The Meat and Poultry Counter	Just a trace
Fruit, Vegetables, Bread and Unfortified Cereals	None

RECOMMENDED DAILY AMOUNT IN WINTER: 5.0 MICROGRAMS

THE B VITAMINS

The third group of vitamins are the B vitamins. Two of the best known, thiamin (vitamin B1) and niacin, help to release energy from the food we eat. They occur in small amounts in a wide variety of animal and plant foods including the husks of cereal grains, and are added to fortified breakfast cereals. They occur naturally in wholemeal bread but have to be added to white.

A shortage of thiamin (B1) and niacin in the diet may lead to tiredness, muscle weakness, loss of appetite and nausea. A severe lack of thiamin results in a disease called beri beri, once prevalent in South East Asia. Rice polishing, removing the outer skin of the rice in order to make white rice, was introduced in the seventeenth century, following which, beri beri, a disease affecting the heart and nervous system, became widespread throughout the region. Fortunately, such an extreme deficiency is unlikely to affect the supermarket shopper in Britain.

Riboflavin (vitamin B2) is another vitamin which helps us to release energy from the food we eat. A large part of the riboflavin in our diet comes from dairy products, such as milk, cheese and yoghurt, but don't worry if you only drink skimmed milk as there is just as much riboflavin in skimmed milk and low fat cheeses as in full fat. It is very sensitive to light so if you buy your milk in bottles keep them in a dark spot, and if you have them delivered, don't leave them too long on the doorstep. If, as in my case, that would mean getting up at 5.30 a.m. every morning, leave a light-proof box on the doorstep for the milkman to drop them in. Eggs are also a rich source of riboflavin and it is found as well in meat, vegetables and cereals. One of the first symptoms of a lack of riboflavin is an increase in our susceptibility to cracks and sores about the mouth.

Now for three lesser known B vitamins, pyridoxine (vitamin B6), biotin and pantothenic acid (vitamin B5). Pyridoxine has many functions in the body, mostly related to the proper use of proteins. It is found in a wide variety of animal and plant foods including liver and wholemeal breads, fish and nuts and fortified breakfast cereals. A deficiency can result in susceptibility to anaemia and skin complaints, muscle weakness and irritability. Biotin has many roles in the body including, once again, helping us to obtain energy from the food we eat. It is found in a wide variety of animal and plant foods. Pantothenic acid (vitamin B5) is also found in a wide variety of foods so again a deficiency is very unlikely to occur. It too helps us to release energy from food.

All of the above vitamins are water soluble and any excess is excreted rather than being stored so we need some every day. Owing to the wide range of foods in which they are found a serious deficiency in Britain is unlikely, but if you want to be really sure of obtaining enough, have a sandwich of Marmite on wholemeal bread! Yes, yeast and wholemeal bread are two of the richest sources of B vitamins so a daily sandwich of Marmite or other yeast extract will put you well on the road to your recommended daily amount! So for that matter will fortified breakfast cereals which, as you will see from the label, have the B vitamins in abundance.

VITAMIN B12

Although it has B in the name, vitamin B12 is so different from the other B vitamins that it really deserves to be put in a class on its own. It has a different kind of function in the body and unlike the other B vitamins we can store it in our liver so we don't need to consume it every day. Also, unlike the other B vitamins, it is not found in fruit, vegetables or cereals. It is often seen along with the other B vitamins on the vitamin list at the side of packets of breakfast cereals, but only because it has been added to the cereals by the manufacturers.

Vitamin B12 either has to be obtained from meat, dairy products or eggs, or from the yeast and seaweed products which also happen to contain it, or from supplements such as those in cereals.

A lack of vitamin B12 is the cause of pernicious anaemia, a kind of anaemia which is fairly common in older people. It is not usually due to a shortage of the vitamin in the diet as such but to a difficulty of absorbing it from the intestines. If taking vitamin B12 pills or eating liver, which is a very rich source, doesn't work, it has to be injected directly into the blood. Because of the limited range of foods in which it occurs and because we are unable to make it ourselves, vegans who avoid not only meat and fish but also dairy products and eggs, are at risk of a deficiency and have to take care that they obtain enough B12. Most now recognise the need for supplements of this vitamin. It is however required in incredibly small amounts. The daily recommended intake is just one millionth of a gram (1 microgram), so a kilogram bag would provide you with enough to last a thousand million days!

If we consume more vitamin B12 than we need, the excess is stored in our livers, so most of us probably have enough in reserve to keep us going for several months even if our diet suddenly became so inadequate that it supplied us with none at all. It is becoming increasingly difficult to suffer from a deficiency of vitamin B12 as it keeps turning up everywhere as a supplement, being added to a whole range of foods which have never before contained it. Those include not only breakfast cereals but fruit drinks, even cans of Heinz spaghetti!

WHERE TO AIM YOUR TROLLEY TO FIND VITAMIN B12 IN THE SUPERMARKET

Product	**Micrograms of vitamin B12 in each 100 gm (3.5oz) of food**
The Meat Counter	
Beef, lamb and pork	2
Rabbit	10
Chicken, dark meat	1
Duck, goose and pheasant	2 to 3
Turkey	2
Bovril	8
The Fish Counter	
White fish	2 average
Fish fingers	2
Oily fish, fresh and canned	4 to 14
Eggs	
Chicken egg (all in the yolk)	2.5 (2 medium eggs)
Duck egg (all in the yolk)	5.4
Milk and Dairy Produce	
Pasteurised milk, full fat, semi-skimmed or skimmed	0.4
UHT milk	0.2
Sterilised milk	0.1
Cheeses, full fat and reduced	1 to 2
Yoghurts	0.2
Ice cream	0.4
Marmite	0.5

SURPRISE SOURCES OF B12: :

Fortified fruit juice drinks	
eg Ribena blackcurrant juice drink	0.5

Fortified breakfast cereals:	
Banana Bubbles, Chex, Coco Pops, Kellogg's Cornflakes, Frosties, Rice Crispies, Nestle Multicheerios, Nesquik, Ready Brek, Weetos	0.8 to 1.0
Heinz spaghetti hoops	0.5

RECOMMENDED DAILY AMOUNT: 1.0 MICROGRAM

FOLIC ACID

Another vitamin, folic acid is found in green leafy vegetables, although potatoes and oranges are also sources. An adequate intake is particularly important during early pregnancy, as there is evidence to suggest that a deficiency may increase the risk of spina bifida in the offspring.

MINERALS

As well as vitamins we also need minerals.

Calcium

By far the most abundant mineral in our bodies is calcium, 99 per cent of which is found in our bones and teeth. Tiny amounts are also needed to allow the blood to clot properly when we injure ourselves and for the proper functioning of the nerves. Children need a lot of calcium for developing bones and teeth as the skeleton increases in size up to the late teens. Even after the growth of the skeleton has stopped, the amount of calcium added to the bone continues to increase for several years after this so that the bones become denser. This can be seen on an X-ray. In our late thirties our bones start to become less dense and weaker, especially in women after the menopause, and in many elderly women the bones are so weak and moth eaten that even quite minor falls can result in fractures. The hip bone is especially vulnerable and a broken hip, known in medical circles as 'a fractured neck of the femur', is a serious hazard of growing old.

So where do we aim our trolley to ensure we get enough calcium to prevent our bones deteriorating? Would it were as simple as that! It would be nice if just increasing our consumption of calcium could keep our bones thick and strong as we get older, but unfortunately the situation is more complicated than this. Bone is not solid calcium as we might expect, but a living structure penetrated by muscle fibres and other living cells. To maintain the complex structure of our bones, regular exercise is essential as well as adequate supplies of vitamin D to ensure that the calcium can be efficiently absorbed from our intestines into our bloodstream.

Milk and dairy products have long been hailed as the richest source of calcium, but plants obviously contain significant amounts of calcium too otherwise how would elephants and rhinoceroses be able to build up and maintain their huge skeletons on a vegetarian diet? Milk, however, is one of the richest sources and semi-skimmed and skimmed milk contain just as much calcium as full fat milk, slightly more in fact. Another rich source is the bones of canned fish which have been softened by the canning process, and also hard water. Full fat and semi-skimmed milk (but not skimmed) and fish also contain the vitamin D which is essential for the calcium to be absorbed properly from our intestines.

Iron

We all know that a lack of iron results in anaemia. This is because iron is needed to make haemoglobin, the substance which gives blood its red colour and which is packed into the red blood cells where its job is to carry oxygen from the lungs around the body to where it is needed. Iron is also part of a similar substance in muscle which ensures that the muscles are kept supplied with oxygen. When we have more iron than we need it is stored in the spleen, kidneys and liver.

The same applies to animals so you can guess what are especially rich sources —kidney and liver and liver products like liverwurst and haggis and blood products like black pudding. Haggis is good stuff with all its iron, vitamins A and B12. No wonder the Scots are so good at throwing telegraph poles around!

There is no shortage of iron in commonly eaten foods – fruit, vegetables and meat all contain reasonable amounts of it. Iron is also added to many breakfast cereals and other processed foods so there is plenty of it around. The problem is that very little of the iron in the food we eat actually passes through the wall of our intestines into our bloodstream where it can be used. The type of iron in meat, fish and poultry is the most readily absorbed but even then we absorb less than a third of what we consume. With the iron present in plants, we are lucky if we absorb 10 per cent, and the amount varies enormously according to what else we happen to eat at the same time. Vitamin C helps us to absorb iron, whereas many other substances like the oxalic acid in rhubarb and spinach bind to it and hold it back. Remember when we were exploring the vegetable section I said that, although spinach has about three times as much iron as most greens, it is in a form which makes it difficult to absorb! Substances in unprocessed bran and the tannins in tea also make it more difficult for us to absorb iron.

To boost our absorption of iron we should follow some of our meals with a glass of orange juice instead of a cup of tea, and include fruits and vegetables rich in vitamin C in as many meals as possible.

Anaemia due to a lack of iron can occur in young people who need it for growth as well as to replace daily losses. Women need more iron than men to replace that lost in blood when they have a period and also need more during pregnancy. Vegetarians tend to be more prone to iron deficiency than people who eat meat since they have to rely on the less readily absorbed type from plants.

Care has to be taken in the use of iron supplements, however, as an excess of iron is of more immediate danger than a deficiency. The small proportion of iron that is absorbed makes it almost impossible to obtain too much from the food we eat, but the highly concentrated source in iron tablets has been responsible for many cases of poisoning in young children. If you take a supplement it should be treated as a medicine and locked securely away. Iron supplements are best taken only on a doctor's advice. It is easy for him or her to tell by a simple blood test whether you need more iron or not, and it is pointless taking a supplement if you don't need it.

THE TRACE ELEMENTS

We also need very small amounts of other minerals including chromium, copper, iodine, manganese, magnesium, molybdenum, selenium and zinc. Their roles are many and varied and the interactions between them so complex that there is considerable dispute about whether supplements are advisable or not. They may upset the balance and do more harm than good. Because we need them in such small amounts they are known as trace elements. Let us start by looking briefly at the best known of the trace elements, iodine.

Iodine

A lack of iodine causes goitre which manifests itself as an enlargement of the thyroid gland in the neck. The gland enlarges in an attempt to compensate for the lack of iodine which is an essential component of one of its hormones. Women are more subject to goitre than men and it is most likely to appear at adolescence or during pregnancy.

Goitre was known in China as early as 3000 BC and was effectively treated by feeding the affected persons with seaweed, which we now know to be rich in iodine from sea water. In parts of the world where there is a tendency to goitre owing to a lack of iodine in the soil, such as Switzerland and Canada, the addition of iodine to salt is required by law. Despite this simple preventative measure, goitre still causes an enormous amount of suffering in certain parts of the world. Worse than the goitre itself, children born of mothers whose thyroid glands are not functioning properly due to severe iodine deficiency (or other causes) may have reduced stature and learning difficulties, the condition known as cretinism.

Goitre due to a lack of iodine is confined to parts of the world where most of the food comes from soils deficient in iodine, but this is not a problem in Britain. Cases of goitre in Britain are not usually due to a simple lack of iodine but to a hormonal imbalance, so anyone noticing that they have a swollen thyroid should see their doctor before taking a supplement.

Zinc

This trace element recently passed through one of those phases which most trace elements pass through at one time or another where it was being hailed as the cure for all our ills. This place has now been taken by selenium which we will talk about later on.

Zinc is used in industry as a coating for galvanised iron, as a component of flashlight batteries and, alloyed to copper, for making brass. In our bodies it has even more uses. A lack of zinc in the diet of children can result in stunted growth and loss of appetite. In adults it is needed for the proper structure of the skin and for wound repair and has been shown to be effective in the treatment of certain forms of acne in zinc deficient persons. A normal balanced diet should provide all of the zinc we need, so if we have any of these symptoms they are much more likely to be due to some other cause than to a lack of zinc. Zinc is present in small amounts in virtually all foods, the richest sources being meat products and whole cereal grains. Zinc is lost when flour is refined, another reason for eating wholemeal bread which contains three times as much of the mineral as white bread.

Cobalt

Although cobalt is an essential mineral we need so little of it that a deficiency virtually never occurs in man. Interestingly it is part of the structure of vitamin B12, and as long as we are getting enough B12 it would be difficult to get too little cobalt.

Magnesium

Magnesium has innumerable functions in the body. We need it along with calcium for the formation of our bones, although only tiny amounts of it are required by comparison with calcium. We also need it for the transmission of nerve impulses along our nerves, and for the movement of muscle. Without it we would be in a bad way, but deficiency only occurs in special circumstances like starvation, severe alcoholism associated with self-neglect, inflammation of the pancreas, or prolonged diarrhoea and vomiting. It is found in almost all foods and efficiently absorbed.

Selenium

Selenium is now hailed as the wonder mineral because of the antioxidant properties it shares with the ACE vitamins. It has attracted a lot of attention in recent years as a result of the suggestion that it may help to protect against cancer and heart disease. It is found in all sea-food and meat and cereal grains. The amount in cereal grains, however, depends on the amount in the soil in which the cereal was grown. Canadian wheat from which a lot of British bread used to be made tended to contain far more selenium than European wheat from which most of our flour is now made so we may be getting less from this source than we used to. The selenium story is so complex that it is difficult to work out with any degree of confidence how much we should be consuming. The problem is that in high doses it is known to be toxic. Animals grazing areas where the soil is rich in selenium can be poisoned by it, especially if they happen to consume the particular kinds of wild plants which have the knack of concentrating it, like, in America, Gray's vetch and woody aster.

At the other extreme, trace element deficiency can be a serious problem in sheep and other domestic animals which spend all of their lives consuming grass from one small area. If the soil is deficient in one or more of the trace elements symptoms of deficiency may arise, and mineral supplements have to be provided by the farmer. People can experience the same problem when all of the food they consume is grown in one small area in deficient soil, but for the supermarket shopper consuming, as he or she inevitably will, a variety of foods grown in different parts of Britain and imported from around the world, problems of trace element deficiency are unlikely to arise. For this reason and because the amount of a trace element in a fruit or vegetable depends so strongly on the amount present in the soil in which it was grown, it would not be particularly helpful to provide a 'Where to aim your trolley' shopping list for trace elements as I did for the vitamins.

CHAPTER 5

Bread and Breakfast Cereals

The World Health Organisation recommends that we should obtain at least half of our energy from starch.

As well as potatoes and other root vegetables, that means eating lots of cereal products such as wholemeal bread, rice, pasta and breakfast cereals like Weetabix, Shredded Wheat, Rice Crispies and Cornflakes. These are all good healthy foods which, like the original cereal grain, are packed with starch, protein and B vitamins, and hardly any fat.

THE WHOLEMEAL BREAD COUNTER

Official Recommendation: The amount of bread we eat (as a population) should be increased by half with wholemeal bread.

One of the best things to eat when you want an energy rich snack is, wait for it, a slice of bread. A loaf of wholemeal bread is packed full of starch for energy, has lots of body-building protein, numerous vitamins and minerals and hardly any saturated fat. Now that the wheat flour used for making bread commercially is supplemented with soya flour, the protein in bread is of an even higher quality than it used to be.

Put some lettuce on your bread, some grated carrot,

slices of apple, half-fat or cottage cheese. Even spread a thin layer of sticky honey, jam or marmalade which, although it might be bad for your teeth, will be much better for you than cake and biscuits. Or what about a banana sandwich? Mash up the banana with a fork, add just a little sugar or some honey and spread it on the bread; delicious!

Just look at all the different kinds of bread we have to choose from nowadays. Not so long ago, it was a choice between white sliced and white unsliced and perhaps Hovis brown. Now we are spoiled for choice with dozens of different breads adorning the shelves of a typical supermarket, almost all of them good, healthy wholemeal. This is clear evidence that tastes can change for the better and that producers and retailers really are capable of responding to the challenge of providing a healthier diet.

It is not that white bread is bad for us. For the small number of people who don't like wholemeal bread it is a far more satisfactory alternative than eating no bread at all. It too is a good source of starch and protein, but wholemeal bread is even better because it is made from the whole cereal grain, whereas in making white flour, the husk, the outer part of the grain, is removed.

The reason this makes a difference is that the husk contains vitamin E, thiamin and other important vitamins. Wholemeal bread would contain more than twice as much thiamin as bread made from white bread were it not a legal requirement in the United Kingdom for white flour to be fortified with added thiamin.

It seems bizarre to remove the vitamins in making white flour and then have to add them again! Thiamin and some other B vitamins are replaced, but there are other vitamins and minerals present in the husk which are not. It is surely far more sensible to eat wholemeal

Cereals and Pulses: The Perfect Match

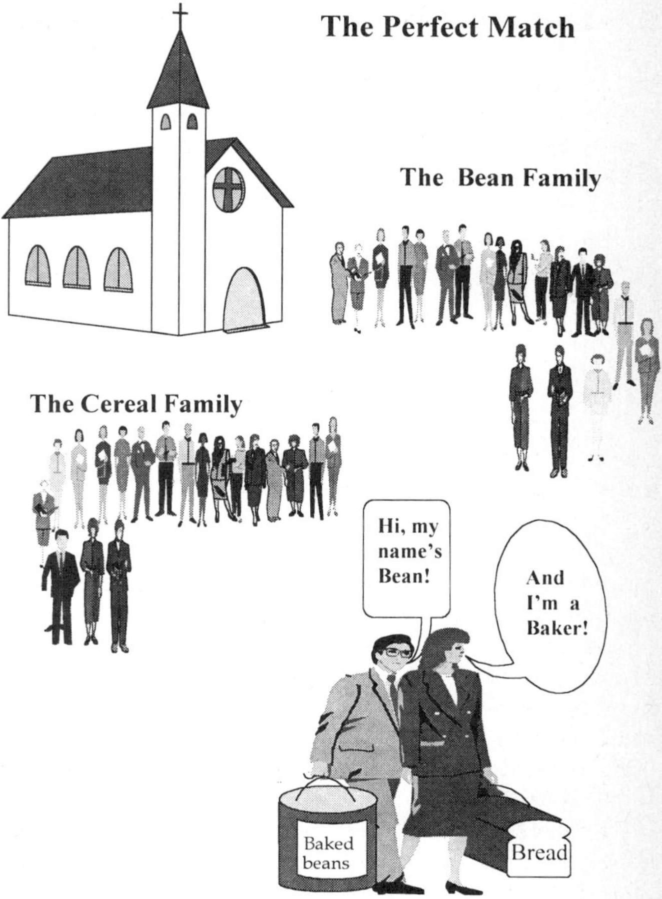

bread with the original thiamin and other vitamins and minerals intact. Then we can be certain that we are getting all the goodness that the cereal grain has to offer.

Quite apart from the vitamins, a further advantage of wholemeal bread is that the husk provides fibre. Not only does this mean less constipation, but fibre in the diet is also believed to protect against bowel cancer, one suggestion being that, by increasing the speed at which waste passes through the bowels, it reduces the length of time that cancer-producing chemicals present in the waste are in contact with the bowel.

Many of these wholemeal breads are so tasty we can eat them by themselves without bothering with any spreads. I often partake of a slice of wholemeal bread when I feel like a snack instead of a biscuit or slice of cake.

A lot of people continue to insist on spreading butter on their bread. This is very much a British tradition. In almost every other country, bread is eaten neat. It seems to be mainly the British who insist on ruining a healthy, fat-free snack by pasting saturated fat in the form of butter all over it. Margarine, the sort that is low in trans-fatty acids is marginally better, but why bother when bread tastes so good by itself?

RICE: THE STAPLE DIET OF MILLIONS

A similar principle, as you will recall, applies to white and brown rice. When white polished rice with the seed coat removed became fashionable in South East Asia, people started to develop a condition called beri beri due to a deficiency of thiamin.

As with wholemeal flour, it is much more sensible to eat whole grain, brown rice rather than the white variety with many of the nutrients polished away.

As there are hundreds of millions of people

throughout the world who eat more rice than anything else, it is obviously a very nutritious, high quality food which can provide the basis of a balanced diet if supplemented with reasonable amounts of vegetables and fruit and pulses. The problem is that in many of the rice-eating countries there often aren't enough of these other foods to go round.

Although many of us in Britain only eat rice in the form of breakfast cereals like Rice Krispies and the occasional pudding, there are enough delicious recipes using rice to enable it to be eaten regularly and provide us with a significant proportion of our energy.

PASTA

Pasta is another rich source of carbohydrate. Macaroni and spaghetti are as rich in starch as the wheat grains they are derived from, and well worth making part of our regular diet.

BREAKFAST CEREALS

Official Recommendation: The amount of breakfast cereals we eat (as a population) should be doubled.

Plain breakfast cereals consist of about 75 per cent starch, which is hardly surprising considering they are made from cereal grains. Because it is from starch that we should be obtaining most of our energy, the expert committees recommend we should double our consumption of them.

A bewildering array of cardboard cereal boxes extends along virtually a whole aisle of the average supermarket. From amongst the more than 200 different cereals to be found on the shelves of the major supermarkets and grocery stores, how do we choose which ones to buy? The simple answer would be to stick to the old favourites – Cornflakes, Rice Krispies, Weetabix, Shredded Wheat, Wheat Puffs and Porridge Oats. It is not that I want to stifle a spirit of adventure, but many of the others have so much sugar added that it would be just as realistic to look upon them as sugar with added cereal. You may think that I am exaggerating until you recall that there are dozens of breakfast cereals like Frosties (basically Cornflakes with sugar) designed to be appealing to children which contain a massive 40 per cent sugar, while almost exactly one half (49 per cent) of a Sugar Puff is sugar.

When choosing a breakfast cereal, check the label on the side of the packet to find out how much sugar it contains and go for the one where the carbohydrate is nearly all starch, and persuade your children to do the same. Well, one can always live in hope! If you have any children around try offering them a box of Wheat Puffs, the sugar-free equivalent of Sugar Puffs, and you may well be surprised at their reaction. I have seen children who have been brought up on sugared cereals find these sugar-free ones such a novelty that they eat them raw like crisps.

Many breakfast cereals also contain large amounts of added salt. As salt contributes to high blood pressure it is best avoided, if not necessarily by children certainly by the elderly and those with a tendency to high blood pressure. For children, choose cereals low in sugar to discourage the development of the sweet and decayed tooth; while middle-aged and elderly people who need to keep their salt intake down, should go for the low salt varieties.

It is with a proverbial pinch of salt, however, that we should take claims made by cereal manufacturers. The side of a packet of Weetos makes interesting reading:

'Weetos contain all the goodness of whole wheat. They also have a delicious chocolate taste, so you know that your children are getting the best of both worlds. An exciting tasty breakfast cereal that is good for them.' Weetos in fact have over seven times as much sugar as the Weetabix made by the same company, but only half as much fibre. The amount of energy is much the same in both products, so wouldn't 'your children' and their teeth and bowels be better off eating Weetabix?

My choice of healthy breakfast cereals from the sugar and salt point of view are listed below. The figures are grams per 100 grams of cereal.

HEALTHY AND NOT SO HEALTHY CEREALS

Type of cereal	**Sugars**	**Sodium**	**Fibre**
Low in sugars AND salt			
Plain Puffed Wheat (Quaker)	0.3	0.0	5.6
Shredded Wheat (Nestlé)	0.7	0.0	10.0
Ready Brek (Weetabix Ltd)	1.7	0.1	8.0
Whole Wheat Flakes (Safeway)	4.4	0.4	10.1
Weetabix (Weetabix Ltd)	4.7	0.3	10.1
Porridge Oats (Quaker)	1.1	0	7
Low in sugars but high in salt			
Cornflakes (Kellogg's)	8	1.1	1.0
Rice Krispies (Kellogg's)	10	1.2	0.7
Special K (Kellogg's)	15	0.9	2.5
High in sugar but low in salt			
Sugar Puffs (Quaker)	49	0	3
Weetos (Weetabix Ltd)	35.9	0.3	5.5
For comparison, some typical cereals high in both sugar AND salt			
Kellogg's Coco Pops	38	0.9	1.5
Kellogg's Frosties	40	0.8	0.6

Many of the sugary breakfast cereals also contain a cocktail of totally unnecessary colourings and flavourings and indigestible plastic toys!

An acceptable compromise is to start with a bowl of the basic, healthy cereal, say a couple of Weetabix, and sprinkle on a few of the sweeter, more colourful cereals. That way the overall sugar content remains lower and we inflict on ourselves a lower dose of colourings and flavourings than if we were to eat the alternative cereals neat.

If we want to be adventurous, there are a few interesting recent additions to the cereal shelves. We can say 'Hello' to cereals like Cheerios in hoop-shaped bites made from a variety of different whole cereal grains – wheat, maize, oats and rice – all in the one packet. They have twice as much sugar as Cornflakes but less than half as much as Frosties, and a limited number of additives, and taste good, so are probably worth a try.

They are called *breakfast* cereals, but a bowl of cereal with semi-skimmed or skimmed milk can be enjoyed at any time of day when we feel like a snack. They are perhaps a bit messy to eat in the office, but at home, no problem! Some cereals like Cheerios and Corn Pops can also be nibbled raw without milk and added to the school lunch box as a healthier alternative to crisps. Although there is more sugar in them than reason dictates, they also contain a lot of starch and vitamins and are very low in fat and so are much better for us than crisps and snack bars.

As well as forming the basis of porridge – what could be better than porridge oats with warm semi-skimmed milk to warm you up on a cold winter's morning? – and a component of the new multi-cereal breakfast cereals, oats are also a component of muesli, another good healthy food we should be eating more of. Oats were once widely grown in Britain for human consumption and were the staple diet of the Scottish population before potatoes came along. Comparatively few oats are grown nowadays, which is a pity because they are a good, nourishing food, with the typical cereal qualities of lots of energy-yielding starch and body-building protein.

WHERE TO AIM YOUR TROLLEY TO KEEP YOUR BOWELS MOVING

Although not quite the universal panacea for all ills our grannies may have had us believe, keeping the bowels moving is highly desirable. Our digestive systems evolved to handle a diet consisting mostly of fruit and vegetables which contains a lot of fibrous material which cannot be digested.

This indigestible waste fibre absorbs water in its passage through the bowel and the increased bulk stimulates the walls of the lower part of the intestine known as the colon, creating the desire to pass stools more frequently, while their softness makes it easier to satisfy this desire. Towards the end of the last century the fibre content of the average diet plummeted as white flours and sugar began to supply most of the carbohydrate content of the diet, replacing the whole grain porridges and breads which had previously been eaten, which in their turn had replaced much of the fruit and vegetables of previous generations. The problem with all of this processed food is that it can be almost completely digested. This may seem a strange thing to say, but what it means is that there is less waste to be got rid of and what there is tends to get stuck because it cannot provide the gentle stimulation of the bowel wall necessary to eliminate it.

This situation is usually automatically rectified on switching to a healthy diet containing lots of fruit and vegetables, and whole grain cereal products, but if we are only just making the switch, let's see how we can speed things along by having a quick whiz along the shelves to see what are the best sources of fibre.

GOOD SOURCES OF FIBRE

	The richest sources of fibre have the most stars
Breakfast Cereals	
Wheat bran	*****
All-Bran	*****
Bran Flakes	*****
Fruit 'n'fibre	****
Muesli	****
Shredded Wheat	****
Shreddies	****
Weetabix	****
Ready Brek	****
The Bread Counter	
Wholemeal bread	***
White bread	**
The Fruit and Vegetable Section	
Beans and peas	***
Raspberries, blackberries, blackcurrants	***
Root vegetables	**
Greens	**
Other fruit	**
Nuts	***

So for regular, readily ejected, satisfying stools eat plenty of fruit and vegetables, especially peas and beans, wholemeal bread and high fibre breakfast cereals. Weetabix is a good source of fibre without the high in fibre taste of some of the other breakfast cereals.

As well as reducing the agony of constipation, and saving a lot of money in laxatives, consuming plenty of fibre may also help to prevent more serious disorders like irritable bowel syndrome, diverticulosis and diverticulitis. 'Divert- What?' Let me explain. This is a condition in which small 'balloons' bulge into the walls of the large intestine and then become inflamed resulting in abdominal pain which can be quite severe. It has been suggested that this happens because in the absence of sufficient fibre the contents of the gut are unnaturally small and hard so that they accumulate and stimulate the gut to contract, but contract as it will it has great difficulty in pushing the beads any further. As a result, the gut builds up too much pressure and in so doing the walls of the gut blow out to form these small protrusions. Diverticula is just a fancy name used by doctors for a small protrusion.

Doctors, you will have noticed, are very fond of using erudite-sounding expressions to impress their patients. A friend of mine was told recently by his doctor that he had chronic idiopathic urticaria. Before you start sending flowers, let us analyse what this means. 'Chronic' means 'you've had it for a long time'; 'idiopathic' means 'of unknown origin'; and 'urticaria' means 'a skin rash'. So what this 'diagnosis' really means is: 'you have got a skin rash which you have had for a long time and we haven't a clue what's causing it.'

But my aversion to unnecessary jargon causes me to digress. These diverticula or protrusions are very common and like the appendix only produce symptoms if they become inflamed, producing the condition diverticulitis. Consuming plenty of fibre may also reduce the prevalence of hiatus hernia and haemorrhoids. It may also reduce the risk of cancer of the colon although we are not absolutely certain of the extent to which fibre protects against these conditions.

What we do know for certain is that adequate fibre in the diet spares us the discomfort of regular constipation so it is worth seeking out for that reason alone.

THE DIGESTIVE SYSTEM

This is as good a point as any at which to look at the digestive system. Our digestive system operates like a complex chemical works which enables our bodies to make use of the food we eat. Digestion starts in the mouth where the action of chewing breaks down food into smaller pieces and the enzymes in saliva start breaking down starch into sugar. That is why starchy foods like bread begin to taste sweet if we chew them for a long time.

When food reaches the stomach digestion is begun in earnest. After being churned up with acid and more enzymes which break down the protein into amino acids, the food is passed out of the stomach into the small bowel. Although called the 'small' bowel it is anything but small being an incredible six metres long, over three times the height of an average person. How surgeons who perform operations on the small bowel ever manage to fit it all back in again beats me! In the small bowel the food is flooded with a succession of more enzymes which break down the food into simple sugars and fats and amino acids, which are absorbed through its walls into the bloodstream.

Undigested food carries on along to the colon where it is attacked by the colonies of bacteria which live there

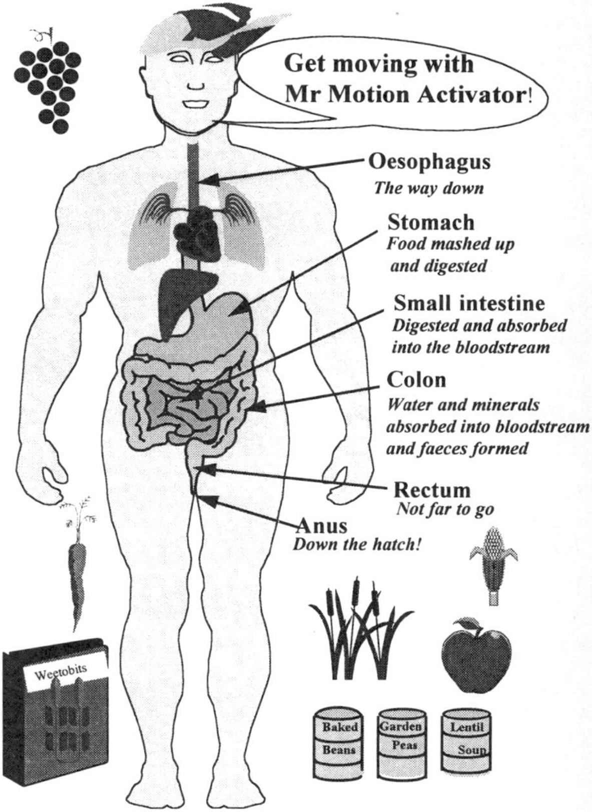
Get moving with
Mr Motion Activator!
Oesophagus
The way down
Stomach
Food mashed up
and digested
Small intestine
Digested and absorbed
into the bloodstream
Colon
Water and minerals
absorbed into bloodstream
and faeces formed
Rectum
Not far to go
Anus
Down the hatch!
Weetobits
Baked
Beans
Garden
Peas
Lentil
Soup

and excess water and minerals are absorbed into the body. The remaining waste is compacted and passed along to the rectum, the last few centimetres of the large bowel, and ejected through the anus. It takes between a day and a half and three days for food to pass right through the body, longer if you are constipated, so if you ever accidentally swallow anything valuable, be patient!

If you decide to change to a high fibre diet do so gradually over a period of months to give your digestive system time to adapt, otherwise you may end up with abdominal discomfort and even diarrhoea which puts you off continuing.

CHAPTER 6

The Meat Counter

Official Recommendation: Reduce (as a population) the amount of processed meat and sausages we eat by a half.

PIGS, SHEEP AND COWS: FIRST CLASS PROTEIN, BUT TOO MUCH SATURATED FAT

Isn't meat good for us then? The answer is: 'like everything else, in moderation.' Meat is an excellent source of first-class protein but many people eat far too much red meat in one form or another. Not content with the Sunday roast, they also shovel down mince, sausages, burgers, luncheon meat and meat pies . You may wonder how we can possibly eat too much meat. After all, human beings have been eating animals for millions of years, so doesn't that mean that meat is a natural food which must be good for us?

The key to this apparent contradiction lies in the fact that the meat we eat today is so very different from the meat our ancestors ate. Our meat comes mainly from three species – sheep, cattle and pigs – not from the wild game that the hunter-gatherers of old consumed.

But why should that make a difference?

The reason is that present-day sheep, cattle and pigs are fat, incredibly fat, compared to their lean wild relatives. Over a quarter of the meat we obtain from these domesticated animals is fat. This is in sharp contrast to the wild game, the rabbits, deer, wild goats and other wild animals, that our ancestors used to eat, which all contained less than five per cent fat. In fact almost all wild animals that live on the land contain less than five per cent fat. Ironically, out of the several thousand species of mammals in the world, the three that we eat most of are the most unhealthy for us.

As a pound of beef or pork contains five times as much fat as a pound of rabbit or venison, to say that people have always eaten meat is a false argument because the meat that people used to eat until a few generations ago was so much healthier than the fat, lamb, beef and pork that is eaten today.

You may wonder why present-day sheep, cattle and pigs are so fat. There are at least two reasons for this. Firstly, it is the result of years of selective breeding. In order to produce meat that's as tender as possible, the animal breeders have repeatedly bred from fatter animals so that in successive generations the animals have become fatter and fatter. Also, before vegetable oils became so readily available in Britain, there was a big demand for fat in the form of lard for cooking, and remember that in the olden days, before we all had electric lighting, fat was highly prized for making candles.

So couldn't the fat just be bred out of them again?

Yes it could be if the incentive were there. A number of agricultural research establishments have been applying their talents towards breeding leaner pigs with some success, but they still have an extremely long way to go to get back down to the wild boar level.

The second reason why they are so fat is that domestic animals are fed so intensively and need to take so little exercise to obtain their food and to keep warm that they naturally become fatter. Over-eating, and under-exercising is the universal recipe for obesity, for pigs as for people.

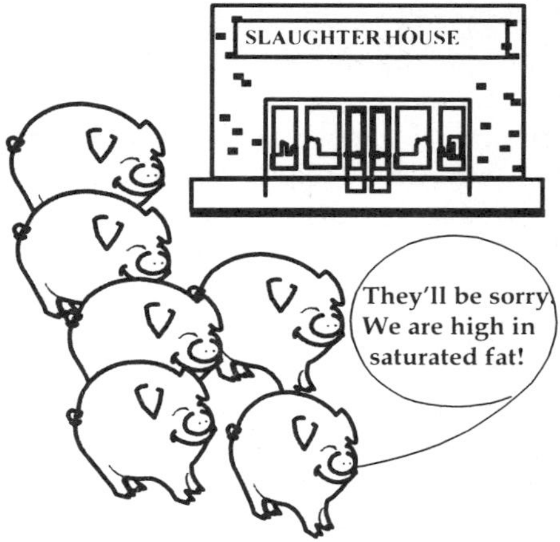

The worst part about it is that much of the extra fat in domestic animals is the unhealthy kind – saturated fat.

Next time you pass by the meat counter in your local supermarket, you will see what I mean about saturated fat. It's oozing from the pork, the lamb, the beef, the sausages, the meat pies, the mince, the corned beef, possibly even the butcher behind the counter if he over indulges in his own product.

Twenty-five per cent is of course the average amount of fat in cattle, pig and sheep meat. At the one end of the range, you can get so-called 'lean' cuts with around 15 per cent fat and at the other, fatty bacon with a massive 40 per cent fat.

Liver is generally considered worth eating in moderation as it is exceptionally rich in vitamin A, vitamin B12 and iron. Haggis incidentally is the heart, lungs and liver of a sheep or deer minced together and mixed with suet, oatmeal, onions, salt and pepper, and then boiled in a skin like that of a sausage. It used to be enjoyed all over Britain, but is now considered a Scottish delicacy. Haggis is an excellent source of iron, vitamin A and vitamin B12 from the heart and liver.

SHOULD WE STOP EATING MEAT FROM CATTLE BECAUSE OF FEARS ABOUT BSE?

Many people have already stopped eating beef and beef products. Some schools have taken beef off their menus altogether, while others have just banned the processed meat like sausages and burgers, but is it really necessary?

The answer to this question is that no-one really knows. There are two main questions to be resolved. Firstly, are infected meat and meat products getting through the checks and being sold for consumption? Most infected animals are spotted on the farm or at auction before they get to the slaughter house but it would be unrealistic to believe that the controls are 100 per cent effective. A small amount of infected meat is bound to get through occasionally, but does it matter?

That depends on the answer to the second question. Can BSE be transmitted to man? The disease can be transmitted to related species, for example between cattle and sheep. It is known that a similar disease in mice can, with difficulty, be transmitted to hamsters. But whether BSE can be transmitted from cattle to man or whether there is any connection between the human equivalent, Kreutzfeld-Jacob disease, and BSE, remains at the time of writing (February 1996), uncertain.

So, sorry, I can't advise you either way.

POULTRY: HIGH IN FIRST-CLASS PROTEIN AND LOW IN UNHEALTHY SATURATED FAT

One thing on the meat counter that does not ooze fat is poultry. Present day poultry meat (excluding the skin) contains very little fat, 5 per cent overall, about the same as wild game like deer and rabbits. That is why it is so much healthier to eat poultry rather than meat from sheep, cattle and pigs which contains on the average five times as much. Why choose red meat when there is chicken right beside it at a lower price per pound? An occasional Sunday joint won't do us any harm, but if we eat meat regularly, most of it should be poultry. Poultry liver, although often discarded, is just as valuable a source of vitamins and iron as sheep or ox liver with the added advantage that it comes free, or used to do so, until the sale of poultry with their giblets was outlawed by the EC on hygiene grounds.

About 450 million chickens are sold each year in Britain for boiling or roasting. The poultry doesn't always have to be chicken however. Pheasants and turkeys with even less fat than chickens are no longer just a Christmas event but are now available all the year round, so they can be eaten whenever we feel like a change. Avoid ducks and geese though, except as a special treat, as they contain a lot more fat than other poultry. Here is a tip: when eating chicken and turkey, if you want to keep your fat consumption really low, don't eat the skin, as that is where much of the fat is. Remove it before cooking if possible and certainly before eating. The white meat has very little fat and what there is, is mostly unsaturated.

The trend is already in the right direction. In Britain today we buy only half as much lamb, beef and veal as we did twenty years ago, while the consumption of poultry has doubled. As for pork, however, consumption has remained much the same.

Chapter 7

With the Animals' Welfare at Heart

If you have a strong concern for the welfare of animals kept for human consumption, your choice of meat may be influenced by the conditions under which the animals are kept.

FREE-RANGE POULTRY

About a third of all fresh poultry purchased by shoppers in France carries the *Label Rouge*, and they are now available in some stores in Britain. The breeds are specially selected for their slower growth rates and meat quality. Fed on a minimum of 75 per cent cereal to enhance their natural flavour with no animal matter, the birds are reared in shaded open-air fields and woodlands for a minimum of 81 days. This is almost twice the life-span of battery-bred birds which are normally slaughtered at 42 days. Such birds are said to have firmer flesh, leaner skin and superior flavour. In France, *Label Rouge* traditional free-range guinea fowl, duck, turkey, goose and quail are also available.

The best-known free-range chickens in British supermarkets, owing to a bit of inspired television advertising featuring actor Dudley Moore, are those stocked by Tesco, which are reared in a hundred square mile forest area in south-west France. As you would expect, free-range chickens are a little more expensive than the battery variety, but not much so. Popping into a local Tesco recently I found them selling fresh, free-range French chickens for 129p per pound, compared with 92p per pound for their battery-bred British cousins, not a lot extra really for a finer taste, even lower fat and a clearer conscience.

Free-range chickens are also available from Marks and Spencer, the expanding town centre frozen food store Iceland and other supermarkets, most of which come from a company in Northern Ireland called Moy Park.

Tesco also sell, all the year round, free-range turkeys from the woods, if not of France, then of York, again with an only slightly higher price tag. Free-range turkeys are now stocked by most supermarket chains although not necessarily in every store.

Most supermarket ducks and geese are factory farmed with the birds kept, although not in cages, still under very restricted conditions. Marks and Spencer and Sainsburys, however, sell free-range ducks and geese in selected stores at least at Christmas. Ducks and geese, as we have already seen, are higher in fat than most poultry and a less desirable buy anyway from a nutritional point of view. Pheasants are lean and, although mostly reared in game farms, spend most of their lives in a fairly natural environment out of doors.

FREE-RANGE EGGS

Aware of the appalling conditions under which battery eggs are produced, many of us are prepared to pay the little extra for free-range eggs. But beware of misleading descriptions of eggs like 'farm fresh'. If the hens are free range, 'free range' they will be called.

BARN EGGS

Under this system, barn hens are kept indoors, often under dreadfully overcrowded conditions, but at least they are not caged so it is a step in the right direction.

CAKE AND OTHER EGG PRODUCTS: FREE-RANGE OR BATTERY?

Unfortunately, when we consume products made with eggs, like cake, we have no control over where the eggs come from, as the manufacturers never seem to reveal the source. Surprisingly perhaps, because to be able to say that their cake was made with free-range eggs – I doubt if at present they ever are, unless you know different — could be a big selling point.

PIGS FOR PORK

Most pigs are reared intensively in specially built pig houses. A high temperature is maintained in these houses to ensure that most of the food being provided automatically from hoppers goes into increasing weight rather than keeping warm. Under this system, neither the sows nor the growing pigs ever go outside. Pigs being fattened for the butcher are usually slaughtered at six months of age if they are being sold for bacon; those going for pork are dispatched some weeks earlier.

The outdoor system of pig production, under which the pigs are kept outside with small corrugated iron huts known as 'arks' for shelter is, however, gaining in popularity. They are allowed to forage for some of their own food and there are generally less health problems than with intensively reared pigs. The disadvantage of this system – for the farmer rather than the pigs – is that the pigs do not reach killing weight so quickly as they do in a warm house.

All Marks and Spencer's fresh pork is now produced

from animals reared by the outdoor system. At Asda, pork labelled 'Conservation Grade' and at Tesco that labelled 'Traditionally Reared Prime Norfolk Pork' is derived from pigs that spend at least part of their lives out of doors. So is the range of pork available from Waitrose labelled 'Traditional English Pork' and Iceland's 'Naturally Reared Prime British Pork'.

Bacon pigs do not, however, have such a healthy lifestyle. Free-range bacon is hard to come by.

CATTLE, FROM MOUNTAIN SIDE TO VEAL CRATE

Like pigs, the range of conditions under which cattle are kept varies enormously, from those which spend most of their days out in the open fields to the veal calves which spend the whole of their lives indoors in heated houses. Most of the veal eaten in Britain comes from places like Holland where the crate system still operates. Food is provided as a soup in water and the temperature kept high so that the calves will keep eating in an effort to obtain the water they need to quench their thirst. Their movements are constrained so that as little as possible of their food is 'wasted' to provide energy for movement, instead of being used to put on weight. Under such an intensive system they are ready for slaughter at between 13 and 20 weeks of age. Although the most intensive crate system is banned in Britain it is still legal for British dairy calves to be exported to Europe, reared in the very system that has been banned here, and then re-imported as veal, a practice which has aroused tremendous opposition from people concerned about animal welfare.

LAMBS – SOON READY FOR THE CHOP

The happy, gambolling lambs you see chasing each other over the hillside appear to fare better except for the fact that they are only allowed to live for about five months by which time they will weigh about 37 kilograms and be ready for the chop. You don't often find mutton (meat from sheep over one year old) in the supermarkets nowadays, as shoppers tend to prefer the smaller, more tender, cuts and farmers prefer not to keep stock over winter if it can be avoided.

VENISON

Deer are farmed in much the same way as cattle, with the animals spending most of their time grazing out of doors. The ecological problem posed by over-stocking of the Highlands – the deer eat the young seedlings and prevent the regeneration of natural woodland – has prompted the Prince of Wales to persuade Safeway stores to stock exclusively wild venison. You can't get much better than that!

NUTRITIONALLY THINK POULTRY!

As the French experience clearly shows that the rearing of poultry under humane conditions to supply the bulk market is a commercial proposition, is there really any good reason why all of the poultry sold in Britain should not be free range? This would make the consumption of poultry rather than beef, pork and lamb, a clear winner from the animal welfare as well as from the nutritional viewpoint.

The only satisfactory answer at present to the animal welfare question is to become a vegetarian, but failing that, certainly from the nutritional point of view, as we approach the meat counter we should think poultry. If it proves impossible to resist the joint of beef, lamb or pork, go for the leanest cuts. The meat section of the 'Seek and Reduce Calorie and Fat Counter' (pages 225–8) is there to help you choose. Avoid the cuts with lots of visible fat and trim off any you can see when you get home. Visible fat is mostly saturated fat so it is well worth removing. Not that any cut of the Fat Three is really lean compared with the athletic leanness of wild game or poultry. Why not save yourself some money by buying a smaller joint, then nip back to the vegetable section for some extra spuds and greens to make up the difference?

It won't do any harm to tuck into a Sunday joint with plenty of veg, or a traditional cooked breakfast once in a while. But only kamikaze eaters should have daily bacon and eggs for breakfast – fat and cholesterol without the fresh vegetables – and the advice must be to avoid as completely as possible meals based on processed red meat like sausages, burgers, cans of luncheon meat and meat pies which all contain masses of saturated fat.

Warming up with a hot dog at the funfair on a cold winter's night won't do us any harm, but if we want to keep our intake of saturated fat down, we certainly don't want to make a regular habit of processed meat.

If you want to find out more about the welfare of the animals sold for food, I can heartily recommend Audrey Eyton's book, *The Kind Food Guide*, published by Penguin in 1991.

CHAPTER 8

The Fat Jungle: The Different Types Explained

'Saturated fats, polyunsaturated fats, essential fatty acids'; it can all become a bit confusing to say the least, so let us see if we can unravel the difference between the potentially harmful saturated fats in red meat and the various kinds of unsaturated fats which in sensible amounts are good for us.

HARMFUL SATURATED FATS AND THE 30 GRAMS PER DAY LIMIT

Firstly, there are the saturated fats that we are constantly trying to avoid which are found in the largest amounts in meat from pigs, cattle and sheep, including processed meats from these animals like sausages and burgers, and in full fat milk and milk products.

An enormous amount of convincing evidence has been gathered by scientists around the world that people who eat large amounts of saturated fat are at much greater risk of developing heart disease than those whose diet is low in saturated fat. In the Mediterranean countries, such as France, Spain, Italy and Greece, where most people eat lots of fresh fruit and most of the fat they eat is unsaturated, there is a very low incidence of heart disease. The World Health Organisation recommends that we should obtain no more than one tenth (10 per cent) of our energy from saturated fat. So, how do we work that out?

In practical terms, it means that if we use 2,700 kcals of energy in a day, about the average for a fairly active man, no more than 270 kcals of that should be from saturated fat. As 1 gram of fat gives us 9 kcals, it is easy to calculate the maximum amount of saturated fat we are allowed to eat. Just divide 270 by 9 to give 30 grams.

If we are active adults let us set 30 grams as our daily limit of saturated fat. Obviously, younger children and people who are less active and, therefore, need less energy should eat less saturated fat.

Thirty, though, is a good, easy number to remember as

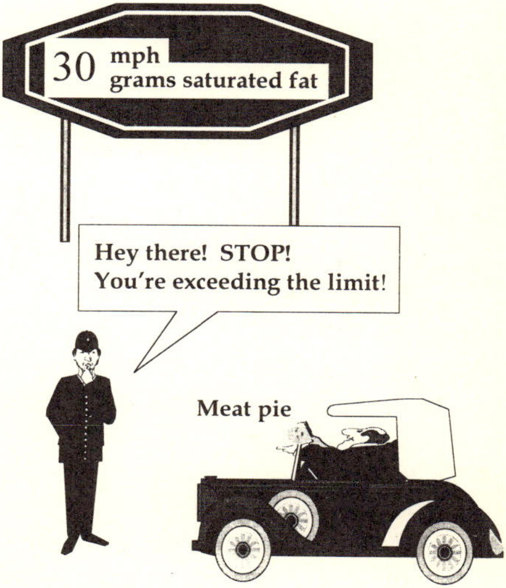

it's the same as the speed limit in town. But remember that the saturated fat limit, like the speed limit, is an absolute maximum. Confining ourselves to 20gm today does *not* allow us to eat 40gm tomorrow anymore than driving at 20mph now would allow us to drive at 40mph later on. An increased risk of obesity now and of heart disease in later life are the penalties for exceeding the *feed* limit. Most of the time, to be on the safe side, we should aim to keep well below the 30 limit whether it's miles per hour or grams of saturated fat per day.

Now for a few yardsticks to help us get a feel for what 30gm looks like.

1 A litre of full fat milk contains about 24gm of saturated fat (40gm total fat).
2 Full fat cheese contains approximately 22gm of saturated fat in every 100gm (34gm total fat).
3 Meat from a pig, sheep or cow contains on the average about 12gm saturated fat in every 100gm (25gm total fat).
4 Poultry, in contrast, (excluding the skin) contains only about 2gm of saturated fat in each 100gm (5gm total fat).
5 For the amount of fat in every 100gm of packaged foods, read the label.

Although 30gm of saturated fat is a very generous – perhaps over generous – limit, millions of people in Britain today consume far more than this. The average person obtains about 16 per cent of his or her energy from saturated fats compared with the recommended maximum of 10 per cent and the situation in Scotland and the North of England is even worse.

Many of those who research the effect of diet on heart disease agree that the damage can begin when we are young, so the earlier we start on a healthy diet the better.

On the other hand, it is never too late to mend our ways, and at whatever age we see the light our heart and circulatory system starts to benefit and is likely to remain healthy longer. If we still drink full fat milk, the simplest way of making a start on reducing our consumption of saturated fat is to switch to semi-skimmed milk.

POLYUNSATURATED FATS: THE KIND WE CAN LIVE WITH

Secondly, there are the polyunsaturated fats. They are found in just about every natural food, plant as well as animal, and in normal amounts are part of a healthy diet. The most concentrated sources of polyunsaturated fat are cooking oils and margarine. If we were to eat a lot of margarine or fried food it would be easy to consume far more polyunsaturated fat than would be usual on a normal diet. As anything in excess may be harmful in the long term, it is therefore a wise precaution not to overdo the cooking oil or margarine.

MONOUNSATURATED FATS: WE CAN LIVE WITH THESE TOO

Thirdly, there are the monounsaturated fats. Like polyunsaturated, monounsaturated fats are found in most plant and animal foods. A particularly rich source is olive oil of which large amounts are consumed in the Mediterranean countries, which happen to have the lowest incidence of heart disease. It would be hasty at this stage to jump in with claims that monounsaturated fat protects against heart disease, but it would probably be safe to assume that it is less likely to damage the heart and circulatory system than saturated fat. So far as is known, monunsaturated fat is not harmful to health in any other way, but everything in moderation!

Rape seed oil is as rich in monounsaturated fat as

olive oil and both these oils are the basis of several new brands of high mono margarines now coming onto the market.

WHERE THE FATS ARE FOUND

To summarise then. There is very little fat in fruit and what there is, is mostly polyunsaturated so we can eat as much of these as we like without worrying about our fat intake. Notable exceptions are the avocado with 14 per cent fat and olives with nine per cent! Cereal grains and hence breakfast cereals and wholemeal bread have around two per cent fat, again mainly unsaturated and healthy. Nuts contain a lot of fat, usually mostly mono and polyunsaturated and can be eaten in moderation but should not be overdone.

Cooking oil and margarine are concentrated sources of both polyunsaturated and monounsaturated fats and can be used in moderation, but again should not be overdone.

Poultry, and wild game like rabbits and deer contain about five per cent fat in all, with roughly equal amounts of the three kinds – a third saturated, a third polyunsaturated and a third monounsaturated. In fish, too, most of the fat is unsaturated. These are the healthy foods, with more unsaturated fat than saturated, that we can eat plenty of.

In contrast, not only do pigs, sheep and cattle contain about five times as much fat as poultry and game, but much of the extra fat is saturated. Full fat milk and cheese, butter and cream also have high levels of saturated fat relative to polyunsaturated. That is why, to avoid overdosing on saturated fat, these foods should only be eaten in moderation.

ESSENTIAL FATTY ACIDS: GOOD FOR THE HEART

But hold on, we haven't finished yet. There is a fourth

type of fat known as essential fatty acids which have attracted a lot of attention in recent years. These are a kind of unsaturated fat. They are known as 'essential' fatty acids because, as we are not able to make them within our own bodies, it is essential to have them in the diet.

The omega-3 essential fatty acids are especially interesting in that they reduce the tendency of the blood to clot and may therefore help to protect against heart attacks. Small amounts are found in most types of food, but oily fish are especially rich in the omega-3 essential fatty acids. This is why people who have had a heart attack are advised by their doctors to eat lots of oily fish to reduce their risk of a recurrence.

Have you got all of that? Remember the saturated fats are the bad guys which clog up your arteries if you eat too much of them and the unsaturated fats the good guys, especially the omega essential kind. So keep an eye on the amount of saturated fat you eat, don't overdo the cooking oil, eat some oily fish or the occasional spoonful of cod liver oil, but otherwise don't worry too much about the unsaturated fats and you will get it about right. Although too much saturated fat is bad for us, a small amount of fat is needed to enable us to absorb the fat soluble vitamins, A, E and D.

HYDROGENATED VEGETABLE OIL AND TRANS-FATTY ACIDS

Oh, no, still haven't we finished yet?

Almost, but there is yet another kind of fat that we should be aware of. You may have seen 'hydrogenated vegetable' oil written on the side of packets of processed food and wondered what it meant. I'll tell you.

Hydrogenated vegetable oil is polyunsaturated vegetable oil which has been treated with hydrogen – hydrogenated – to convert some of the polyunsaturated fat into a kind of saturated fat called trans-fatty acids.

Why ever would anyone want to change healthy polyunsaturated fat into unhealthy saturated?

The answer is: to make the vegetable oil solid at room temperature. Vegetable oil is liquid because it contains mainly polyunsaturated fat, whereas butter is solid because it contains mainly saturated fat.

MARGARINE AND OTHER LOW FAT SPREADS

Margarine is made from vegetable oils by hydrogenating them to convert some of the unsaturated fats into saturated fat so that the margarine is solid at room temperature. Although margarine still has much of the unsaturated fat of the vegetable oil, the saturated ones that have been created chemically are at least as bad for us as those in butter.

The take-home message is that margarine is preferable to butter, but we still need to go easy on it. Always read the labels and choose those margarines with the smallest amount of trans-fatty acids. Unfortunately many brands still fail to provide this vital information but we can easily express our disapproval by not buying them.

What level of trans-fatty acids should we be aiming for? Well, Flora Extra Light has got its trans-fatty acids down to 0.4g in every 100g, so there is no need to buy margarine which contains more than that.

The current trend is for the manufacturers of healthy margarines to reduce the levels of polyunsaturates in favour of monounsaturated which are now considered to be healthier than polyunsaturated. The two cooking oils with the highest proportion of monounsaturated are olive oil and rape seed oil (the one that produces all of those bright yellow flowers which adorn the fields in spring, producing clouds of pollen which gets up some people's noses).

Margarines which are made from olive oil are generally recognisable by their name, for example, Tesco's *Olive* Gold and Heinz Weight Watchers *Olivite*. Manufacturers who use rape seed oil clearly have an identity crisis. St Ivel Rape sounds like a horror headline in a local newspaper so, not surprisingly, St Ivel have opted to call their rape seed oil margarine simply MONO.

Margarine is naturally a good source of vitamin E because the oils it is made from are rich in it, and it is also supplemented with vitamins A and D by the manufacturers to make sure that we do not miss out on these vitamins by eating margarine instead of butter.

If we are calorie counting we should remember that standard margarine contains a similar number of calories to butter, about 740 per hundred grams, but there are as many half fat (and therefore half calorie) varieties on the shelves as there are standard and even a few one third fat varieties. To reduce the fat content of margarine it is necessary for the manufacturers to add water, so the low fat varieties are best for spreading on your bread rather than for cooking. In one way the low fat spreads are not such good value, as much of what you are buying is water. But on the other hand, if you recognise the need to limit your fat intake, and the water allows you to do that while still providing the margarine taste you want, so much the better.

THE LOW FAT SPREAD DILEMMA

	(The type of fat in grams per 100g (3.5 oz))				
	Saturated	**Mono unsaturated**	**Poly unsaturated**	**Trans**	**Total fat**
The low total fat, low trans-group eg Flora Extra Light (sunflower oil)	9	10	20	0.4	39

The high mono-group eg St Ivel MONO (rape seed oil)	11.5	35.0	14.7	Not stated	75

Which of these two groups is best for us? The first group of margarines of which Flora Extra Light is an example are low in total fat and very low in trans-fatty acids, but if you believe that a high ratio of mono to other fatty acids is a good thing you might go for other group of margarines of which an example is St Ivel Mono. The debate still rages. You pays your money and takes your choice.

The situation is rendered even more complex by the recent introduction of margarines containing fish oils which may confer extra benefits.

COOKING OILS

Rich in Polyunsaturated and Monounsaturated Fats and Vitamin E

Over the last few years, this zone has grown and grown. Not so long ago, nearly everyone used either lard or, if they were well off, butter for cooking so, every time they cooked or baked anything, they added masses of saturated fat to it. Fortunately, today there is an amazing variety of vegetable oils to choose from – sunflower oil, corn oil, rape seed oil, ground nut oil, grape seed oil and olive oil, for general cooking and numerous others like walnut oil, sesame oil, and safflower oil used more sparingly to impart special flavours.

The great advantage of vegetable cooking oils over butter and lard is that although they consist entirely of fat most of it is the unsaturated, acceptable kind.

The only common exceptions to the rule are coconut oil in which 90 per cent of the fat is saturated, followed by palm oil, but these can easily be avoided. Cooking oils all have the same amount of fat and the same number of calories, but what they differ in is the relative proportions of the different kinds of fat.

In olive oil, grape seed and rape seed oil, two-thirds of the fat is monounsaturated, while in most of the other vegetable oils two-thirds of it is polyunsaturated. People living on a Mediterranean-type diet consuming a fair amount of olive oil, tend to have lower levels of blood cholesterol and heart disease than people elsewhere consuming a similar amount of total fat. This has led to the suggestion that we should concentrate on those cooking oils with relatively high levels of the monounsaturated fats, like olive oil and rape seed oil. It is not, however, clear whether the monounsaturated fats have a positive beneficial effect on the heart or whether it is the lower proportion of saturated fat which is responsible, or indeed whether most of the benefit is derived from the large amount of fresh fruit which the same people tend to eat. Whatever the explanation, the unsaturated fats of cooking oils are undoubtedly much better for us than the saturated fat of butter or lard, or the trans-fatty acids of margarine.

Sometimes you see vegetable oils described on the label as 'cold pressed'. What does that mean? Cold pressed means that all of the oil has been obtained simply by pressing the seeds, without it being extracted by chemical means. It's a bit more expensive because less oil is obtained from the seeds than by extracting chemically, but it's more natural, has more of the original taste, and there is no danger of it being contaminated by the chemicals used in the other type of extraction process, so you may prefer it.

But we don't want to overdo the cooking oil either, even though it is mostly unsaturated. Always use the least you can get away with. It is also important to remember not to keep on re-using the same old oil, as with repeated use unpleasant chemicals can build up.

The take-home message then is that for frying, we should use a small amount of fresh vegetable oil, preferably cold pressed; never butter or lard. Having said that, it is better to grill, boil or microwave, or use non-stick frying pans, rather than fry, anyway, then we don't add extra fat of any kind.

Now for a word of warning. Just because it says on the label that a product contains *vegetable* fat doesn't necessarily mean that it is good for us. Remember what we said about vegetable oils being hydrogenated for making margarine, a process in which the oils are treated with hydrogen to change the polyunsaturated fat into trans-saturated fatty acids. Once vegetable oil has been hydrogenated, it becomes as bad for us as saturated animal fat and should be avoided as far as possible.

NUTS

Like turkeys, fresh nuts used to be a special Christmas treat, but now they too are available from one country or another all the year round. Look at the variety we have in most supermarkets — peanuts, almonds, hazelnuts, walnuts, cashew nuts, Brazil nuts – either in their shells ready for the nutcrackers or shelled in plastic bags ready for eating.

But are nuts good for us? My reply to that would be 'Yes, in moderation'. At various times and places in the past, hazelnuts have formed a significant part of the diet of country dwellers. Because they are from plants we might expect them to be very low in fat but in fact nuts contain more fat than almost anything else, even more than pork and beef, typically between 40 per cent and 70 per cent by weight, so you can see why I said they should be eaten in moderation.

But as nuts are from plants, doesn't that mean that most of their fat is polyunsaturated or monounsaturated, the kind that it is all right to eat, and not the saturated fat of sausages and burgers which blocks up your arteries?

That is mostly true but there is one very big exception, and I mean big. A coconut contains 10 times more of the harmful saturated fat than healthy unsaturated. The same applies to the desiccated coconut sold in bags for sprinkling on cakes. By all means, go ahead and tuck into the coconut you win at the fairground but don't make them a regular part of your diet, not that you are likely to!

At the opposite extreme, walnuts, hazelnuts and almonds have ten times more unsaturated fat than saturated and can be eaten in moderation. Peanuts, with four times as much unsaturated as saturated, are somewhere in between.

Sunflower seeds are a delicious alternative to nuts. They taste just like nuts but with a softer texture and, what is more, are incredibly cheap, about a third the cost of a similar weight of crisps.

A word of warning though about nuts. Never eat mouldy nuts, especially not mouldy peanuts as they can be contaminated with a kind of mould which produces aflatoxins, substances which are known to give rise to specific types of cancer when fed to animals.

CHAPTER 9

The Dairy Counter

Official Recommendations: No change in total milk consumption, but whole milk to be replaced with semi-skimmed, except for children under the age of two years.

FROM THE COW TO THE CUSTOMER

Modern dairy cows that have been specially bred for their milk yield, can produce enough milk to fill around 15 one-litre supermarket cartons every day for up to ten months after calving.

Imagine you are standing in a parlour that is fitted with automatic milking machinery. The herdsman or herdswoman, standing in a pit in the centre of the herringbone parlour is washing the udders of each group of cows as they take up their positions, then attaches the teat cups to their teats.

The machine, operated by a vacuum pump, draws the milk from the udders in a gently sucking action that imitates that of a suckling calf.

The milk flows from the teat cups into a container that measures the amount of milk taken from the cow. It then flows through some other pipes into a large refrigerated storage tank next door where it is kept cool until it is collected.

The cold milk will be collected by tanker later in the afternoon and taken to the company's dairy where it will be tested for bacteria, checked to make sure it does not contain too much antibiotic and other contaminates and the amount of fat and protein measured. It will then be heat-treated to kill the micro-organisms that cause milk to turn sour, so that it lasts longer, and then packed in cartons.

So, after all this trouble has been taken to keep us supplied with milk, is it good for us, or is it slowly poisoning us?

THE VIRTUES OF MILK : PROTEIN, CALCIUM, AND VITAMINS, ESPECIALLY A AND D

Milk has always enjoyed a very healthy image, and people have been encouraged to drink it. During the Second World War, meat and other food was scarce and there was a fear that people might not be getting enough protein. Milk was the answer as it was a cheap source of protein and was produced on British farms. It was provided for all school-children during the War and in 1944 an Education Act made free school milk compulsory. As well as top quality protein, milk also contains calcium for building healthy teeth and bones and milk sugar for extra energy, as well as significant amounts of several important vitamins including riboflavin, vitamin B12, and vitamins A and D.

In the last few years, however, its image has become tarnished as we have come to recognise the dangers of too much saturated fat.

So, how much fat does milk contain? Four per cent. That may not sound a lot, but it soon adds up if we drink large amounts of milk. A pint of *full fat* milk contains just over 20 grams of fat, about two thirds of it saturated, so if we were to drink a pint a day that alone would take us halfway towards our daily maximum saturated fat allowance of 30 grams.

So should we stop drinking full fat milk, then?

Definitely, but with the emphasis on the *full fat*. DON'T STOP DRINKING MILK.

OUT WITH THE FULL FAT MILK AND IN WITH THE SEMI-SKIMMED

Just change to semi-skimmed which contains only half the amount of fat of whole milk. People have been changing to semi-skimmed milk since the early Eighties, and more than half of the milk sold in our supermarkets is now semi-skimmed, a clear sign that people do care about what they eat and drink.

But what about the protein, sugar, calcium and vitamins? Won't we lose half of these as well when we switch to semi-skimmed milk?

Not at all, that's the beauty of it. The process used for removing half of the fat leaves the protein, sugar and calcium intact. The levels of most of the vitamins stay the same too with the exception of the fat soluble vitamins A and D which are reduced by about two thirds, but as we saw in the vitamin section there are plenty of alternative sources of both of these vitamins so there is no need to worry on this score. Some semi-skimmed milk, like that sold by Marks and Spencer's, is fortified with vitamins A and D so that it contains as much as full fat milk.

And what about the energy?

Half of the energy in full fat milk comes from the sugar and protein, so removing half of the fat doesn't make that much difference.

Milk, therefore, is still a healthy food and we can carry on drinking it but we should always make certain that the milk we are drinking is semi-skimmed. If you drink a lot of milk, say more than a pint a day, why not consider making the second and third pints skimmed milk, which contains hardly any fat at all?

Skimmed milk contains just as much protein, sugar,

Healthy Eating
VIRTUALLY FAT FREE

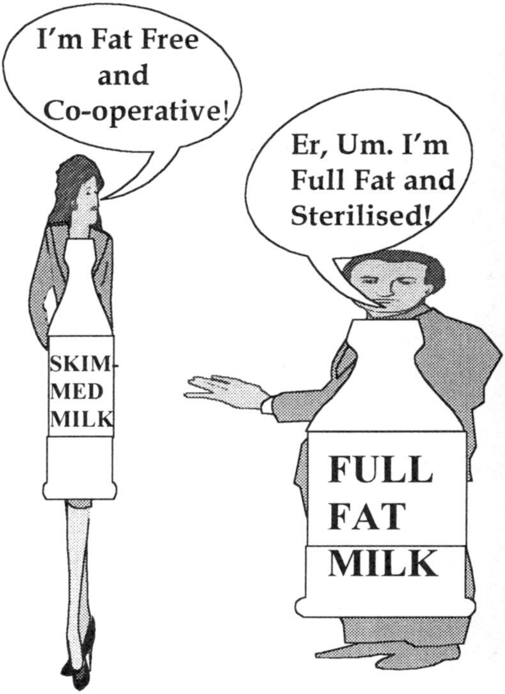

calcium and most of the vitamins of full fat and semi-skimmed and is still excellent body-building stuff. The only things it lacks are vitamins A and D which you can get a daily shot of by making the first pint of the day semi-skimmed or by referring to the vitamin section to find the alternative sources. The really important thing to remember is never to drink full fat milk if you can help it.

This should also mean at school.

Up to the age of two years the expert advice is that children should continue to receive full fat milk, but by the age of five they should be drinking semi-skimmed. Despite this government advice, many children have full fat milk forced on them every day at school. That is something parents of such children should complain about. Nutrition experts all agree that children today are consuming far too much saturated fat, so the schools should never be pushing full fat milk. The milk handed out at break time should always be semi-skimmed. Or at the very least children should be provided with a choice.

SHEEP AND GOATS' MILK

Goats' milk and occasionally sheep's milk are available in some supermarkets. Are they any better for us than cows' milk? Only for people who are allergic to cows' milk. On the plus side they tend to contain more vitamin D than cows' milk, but on the minus side they contain a lot more saturated fat, about half as much again. As the semi-skimmed and skimmed varieties are rarely available, we are as well sticking with cows' milk.

SOYA MILK

This is not milk at all but a milk substitute made from soya beans which may be used by people allergic to cows' milk and by vegans. It has a similar amount of fat as semi-skimmed milk but most is unsaturated.

CHEESE

The problem with fresh milk, as you well know, is that it very soon goes off, so men and women of old devised a clever way of preserving it. They invented cheese making. The aim of this ancient art is to take all the nutrients from the milk and leave the water behind. The cheese is made by adding rennet, which comes from the digestive juices of a calf, to warm milk. This causes the milk to separate into the solid curds containing the nutrients and the liquid whey which is drained off. The type of curd produced depends on the amount of rennet used, and the quality and temperature of the milk. This, together with the different techniques for converting curd into cheese, determines the finished product. At the one extreme we have Cheddar, which is very hard, and at the other, cottage cheese, which is very soft.

As a young friend pointed out the other day, there is one kind of cheese that is made backwards. Can you guess what it is? The answer is Edam. Think about it!

OUT WITH THE FULL FAT CHEESE

Cheese contains roughly the same nutrients as milk but is much more concentrated so, as you can guess, that made from full fat milk contains far too much saturated fat, and should be consumed with caution. A hard cheese like Cheddar contains just over one third fat, even more than pork or beef, so to avoid overdosing on saturated fat it is important to go easy on full fat cheese. Edam has slightly less fat, about 25 per cent. Like the milk it is made from, cheese is a good source of protein so we don't want to stop eating it from a nutritional point of view, apart from which it tastes good. So what do we do? There is a simple solution; switch to half fat and cottage cheese.

IN WITH THE HALF FAT AND COTTAGE CHEESE

Not surprisingly, cheese made from semi-skimmed or skimmed milk contains less fat.

Made from skimmed milk, cottage cheese has only around four per cent fat while still retaining all the protein and calcium of full fat cheese. It does taste somewhat different from ordinary cheese though, so if it's the real cheesy taste you crave, seek out the varieties made from semi-skimmed milk. These have less than half the fat of Cheddar, about 14 per cent, but just as much protein, calcium, vitamin B12 and riboflavin. Most supermarkets already stock two or three kinds of half fat cheeses but be prepared to search for them as they tend to get lost amongst all the other, less healthy varieties. Supermarkets are always ready to respond to demand, and as more and more of us opt for the half fat cheeses they will gradually take over from the full fat just as semi-skimmed milk has displaced full fat milk and wholemeal bread is taking over from white bread.

Why buy full fat milk or full fat cheese when there is the half fat variety with the same amount of first-class protein, calcium and most of the vitamins sitting next to it on the same shelf?

BUTTER, THE ULTIMATE IN UNHEALTHY SATURATED FAT

Butter is solid fat, two thirds of it artery clogging, saturated fat. To make matters worse most butter contains large amounts of added salt. And to think that butter once had a healthy image! If consumed at all, it should be taken in small amounts only. One in ten people in England still use butter or lard for cooking and one in five spread butter or hard margarines (with a high proportion of saturated fat) on their bread. Why, when there are so many healthier alternatives?

But perhaps I am being a little unfair. Butter does contain calcium and vitamins A and D. But it is better by far to get these nutrients from semi-skimmed milk, half fat cheese, and fish, or make the vitamin A in our own bodies from the beta-carotene present in carrots and other vegetables. With far more protein and less fat, other dairy products are much more nutritious than butter.

DOUBLE CREAM

Everything I have to say about butter applies equally to double cream. It is hard to understand how anyone can spoil such a beautiful, healthy fruit as a strawberry by drowning it with dollops of saturated fat in the form of double cream as they do at Wimbledon. Give me the strawberries; you can keep the cream!

After changing from full fat to semi-skimmed milk, not many of us are going to be so perverse as to buy cartons of double cream, but it is still on the supermarket shelves. Just ignore it and perhaps it will go away!

YOGHURT: LOW IN FAT, HIGH IN CALCIUM AND VITAMINS

Yoghurt has a very healthy image. It is nutritious, convenient and there is no problem is persuading children to eat it, but is it as good for us as we imagine it to be?

Yoghurt has a lot going for it. It is made by adding a culture of special harmless bacteria to warm milk. This is kept warm for a few hours to allow the bacteria to multiply and convert the sugar in the milk into lactic acid which partially curdles and thickens the milk and gives it its tangy taste. Being made from milk it is a good source of first-class protein, calcium, vitamin D and other vitamins .

Bio yoghurts contain one or two extra types of bacteria which give these yoghurts a milder, less acidic taste. The bacteria added are usually *Bifidobacterium bifidum* and *Lactobacillus acidophilus* which should be alive and present in their millions when the yoghurt is eaten. Whether or not we ever eat yoghurt, these harmless bacteria are present naturally in our gut where they help to suppress the growth of harmful bacteria such as *Salmonella* and yeasts like *Candida*, the cause of thrush. It has therefore been suggested that ingesting these bacteria in yoghurt may be to the advantage of people whose natural inmates have been depleted by antibiotics or severe diarrhoea.

Despite being made from milk, most supermarket yoghurts, usually described as 'low fat', have only about a gram of fat in each 100ml, not enough to bother about, and many have as little as a tenth of a gram in a tub. Compare that with a typical small (33g) packet of crisps which will contain about 12 grams of fat, a hundred times as much, and you can see just how much healthier it is to get into the habit of having a yoghurt as a snack. The price is much the same too. Even yoghurts described as 'Thick and Creamy' often have no more than the 4 per cent fat of full fat milk; Muller do one at 4 per cent, and Asda at 3 per cent.

A 200 gram tub of a typical low fat yoghurt actually contains as much energy as a packet of crisps, so it will keep us going for as long, secure in the knowledge that the energy is being derived, as it should be, from carbohydrate and protein, and not from saturated fat.

A word of warning though. You may find lurking around the shelves one or two brands often referred to as Greek style yoghurts which have a lot more fat, typically around 10 per cent, just over half of it saturated so a typical 150g pot will provide us with 8g saturated fat.

Worse still, Natural Greek style yoghurts are often sold in giant 500ml pots rubbing shoulders with pots of Natural Low Fat Yoghurts, so beware. Watch out too for chocolate mousse. They may look innocent enough sitting there in their little plastic pots amongst the yoghurts but they have even more fat than Greek style yoghurts. Thirteen per cent, over half of it saturated, is typical of the little blighters, although there are some lower fat options appearing on the shelves.

Natural low fat yoghurt is just fermented milk but flavoured yoghurts may contain all manner of things to add flavour, sweetness and texture.

Sugar is the main additive to be found in yoghurts. The best have no sugar apart from what was already present in the milk, nor do they have any other additives. Many have no added sugar, but do sport artificial sweeteners, flavouring, thickeners and other additives. Many other yoghurts, particularly those meant to appeal to children, have about three level teaspoonfuls of sugar (15g), in each 150g pot as well as flavourings, colourings and other additives, the identity of which will be revealed if we read the label. If you are a vegetarian you will need to avoid those containing gelatine as a thickening agent.

Working on the premise that while large amounts of sugar are undesirable, large amounts of saturated fat may be deadly in the long term, a small amount of extra sugar in our yoghurt, as in our breakfast cereal, is perhaps an acceptable price to pay if it means that we and our children will actually eat the low fat product.

ICE CREAM: WHY NOT TREAT YOURSELF OCCASIONALLY!

All of those plastic tubs of dairy ice cream and choc-ices piled up in the freezer are almost too tempting to resist.

Shall we lean over and have a look, or shall I be a spoilsport and say 'move along there, please' remarking that ice cream is terribly bad for us as it contains far too much saturated fat and eggs?

That is partly true. Ice cream sometimes does contain too much fat. Indeed anything called 'dairy' ice cream must contain at least five per cent milk fat – the average is nearly twice that – and no vegetable fat. Luxury dairy ice creams often contain 15 per cent or more milk fat, two thirds of it the harmful saturated kind, a luxury we can well do without! Just imagine, a litre tub of luxury dairy ice cream contains as much fat as four litres (around eight pints) of full fat milk! Hopefully we wouldn't scoop down a litre in one go, but some people might. If they did they would consume 100 grams of saturated fat at one sitting which is over three times the recommended daily maximum limit of 30 grams.

Choc-ices tend to have the most fat. Wall's Magnum for example has 18 per cent and Wall's Feast 24 per cent!

So long as an ice cream does not describe itself as 'dairy' it can be made with vegetable fats, around a half of which are usually the saturated kind, a bit better than the two thirds of 'dairy' ice cream, but traditional ice creams of this kind still often contain far too much fat.

All is not lost, however, because as soon as we start rummaging through the freezer we will come across a number of low fat varieties which taste just as good as the high fat. The lower fat ices typically have around four per cent fat. Although that is as much as in the whole fat milk that I keep saying we should avoid, so long as we resist the temptation to scoff it by the pint, and confine ourselves to the amount we would get in a cone from an ice cream vendor, let us by all means treat ourselves occasionally.

Even better are the frozen desserts like Wall's 'Too

Good to be True' or Safeway's 'Virtually Fat Free, frozen desserts'. They look and taste very similar to conventional ice cream and as their names suggest have hardly any fat at all, less than half a gram in every 100 grams, not enough to bother about. A bigger helping of these would be permissible. All ice creams and frozen desserts, even Too Good to be True, contain a lot of sugar but, just this once, who cares!

CHAPTER 10

Eggs and Cholesterol

A single hen of one of the strains that have been bred specially for their egg-laying ability can lay enough eggs to provide the supermarket shopper with a fresh half dozen carton almost every week of the year. With eggs in such abundant supply this raises the question, 'Are eggs good for us?'

Some people are put off buying eggs because of their fears about cholesterol. This is a pity because egg whites are an excellent source of almost pure, first class protein. *We can eat as many* COOKED *protein-packed whites as we like.*

EAT MORE PROTEIN-PACKED WHITES: BUT LIMIT THE CHOLESTEROL-RICH YOLKS

It has been known for many years that people with exceptionally high levels of cholesterol in their blood are at higher risk of developing heart disease. Although consuming large amounts of cholesterol does not necessarily increase the amount in the blood, the evidence suggests that too much cholesterol in the diet, on top of the cholesterol which we make ourselves in our livers, may increase the risk of heart disease in people who also eat too much saturated fat.

There is no need to be put off buying eggs altogether because of concerns about cholesterol because, as all of the cholesterol is in the yolk, not eating the yolks is a simple way round the problem.

If you have just two or three eggs a week, by all means go ahead and eat the whole thing. The occasional yolk won't do you any harm and it also contains some useful vitamins. Whole eggs are a good source of vitamin B12 for people who are allergic to dairy products. But if you have eggs every day for breakfast, and especially if you get two eggs for breakfast, it might be wise just to tuck into the protein in the whites, and leave at least one out of every two yolks for the cat. This becomes more important the more saturated fat you eat.

All eggs contain large amounts of cholesterol, including roe, fish eggs being no exception. Duck eggs contain twice as much cholesterol as hens' eggs, not only for the obvious reason that they tend to be bigger, but also because they contain nearly twice as much cholesterol per 100 grams.

BEWARE OF THE HIDDEN CHOLESTEROL IN CAKES AND PASTRIES

The saturated fat and cholesterol in bacon and eggs are obvious, but in other foods, especially cake, they lurk unseen. It is all too easy to forget that cake, unless baked by an exceptionally health conscious cook, is made from the lethal combination of whole eggs and masses of saturated fat, and is as bad for us as regular bacon and eggs.

OTHER SOURCES OF CHOLESTEROL

What other food contains cholesterol?

Cholesterol is totally absent from cereals, fruit and vegetables and is found only in foods originating from animals. One of the few foods that contains more cholesterol than eggs is brains but few people eat brains nowadays owing to concerns about BSE, the so-called 'mad cow's disease'.

Cholesterol and Saturated Fat: The Lethal Combination

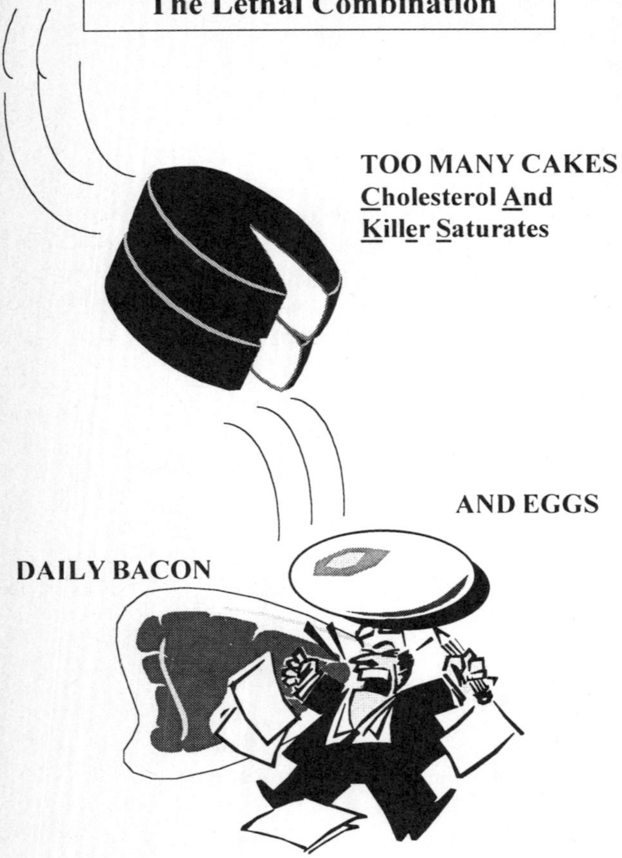

Liver and kidneys also contain about as much cholesterol as the same weight of eggs, but liver of all kinds, including that of poultry, is such an excellent source of vitamin A, vitamin B12 and iron that despite its cholesterol it is still worth eating from time to time. Bird's Eye Boil in the Bag Liver and Onion is one convenient source. Add a packet of frozen vegetables for a quick tasty meal that requires only boiling water.

Butter too has nearly as much cholesterol as the same weight of eggs and masses of saturated fat to boot. Other dairy products like milk and cheese also contain cholesterol. Semi-skimmed milk, however, has only half as much as full fat milk and skimmed milk has even less. Similarly, half fat cheese has only half as much cholesterol as full fat cheese and cottage cheese has very little. Meat of all kinds, whether red meat, poultry or sea-food, also contain a significant amount. The more meat and dairy products we eat, the wiser it is, therefore, to avoid the extra cholesterol in egg yolks and butter.

As meat from wild game such as deer and rabbits only contains about one fifth as much fat as meat from pigs, sheep and cattle, does the same apply to cholesterol? Unfortunately, it doesn't. Meat from wild game has just as much cholesterol as that from domesticated animals.

CHOLESTEROL PLUS SATURATED FAT – THE LETHAL COMBINATION

If that is the case, as our ancestors have been eating eggs and wild game for millions of years, why have we suddenly decided that cholesterol is bad for us?

As we have already remarked, it seems to be not so much the cholesterol by itself which is the problem but its combination with too much saturated fat.

WHERE CHOLESTEROL LURKS IN THE SUPERMARKET

	mg cholesterol per 100g (3.5 oz) food	
Eggs		
Whole chicken eggs	385	(all in the yolk, 190mg in a grade 6 egg)
Whole duck eggs	680	(all in the yolk)
Omelette and quiche	140-360	
The milk and dairy counter		
Full fat milk	14	(about 80mg in a pint)
Semi-skimmed milk	7	(about 40mg in a pint)
Skimmed milk	2	(about 11mg in a pint)
Double cream	130	
Butter	230	
Full fat cheese	70 to 115	
e.g. Cheddar cheese	100	
Reduced fat cheese	43	
Cottage cheese	13	
Dairy vanilla ice cream	31	
The meat counter		
Liver and Kidney	400	
Most meats	Typically around 100	
Sausages	50	
Fish	Typically around 50	
Cod roe	500	
Herring roe	700	
The biscuit section		
Chocolate digestives	51	(about 6mg per biscuit)
Plain digestives	41	(about 5mg per biscuit)
Shortbread	74	

Cakes	Typically around 100
Buns, pastries and puddings	Typically around 50
Chocolate	30

Our hunter-gatherer ancestors may have eaten the eggs of wild birds occasionally when they could get hold of them (presumably fertilised eggs with the developing chick inside them, yuk!), but they certainly would not have had fat bacon and eggs for breakfast every morning, nor would they have stuffed themselves full of cake and pastry made from eggs and butter.

CHAPTER 11

The Fish Counter

Official Recommendation: oily fish intake to double.

FISH FOR TOP-QUALITY PROTEIN, VITAMINS AND THE OMEGA-3 ESSENTIAL FATTY ACIDS

White fish

Fish is one of the healthiest of foods. White fish is high in first-class protein, and low in calories and fat, so it provides a perfect alternative to other sources of animal protein like beef. Cod and haddock at the moment tend to be fairly expensive owing to a reduction in stocks due to over fishing, but other slightly less familiar, but no less nutritious, kinds like coley, hake and whiting are often available at a lower price.

The familiar flatfish such as plaice and lemon sole which live on the sea bed are as rich in protein and low in fat, and just as easy to prepare as their vertical relatives. They can be grilled or, better still, steamed between two plates over boiling water. If the boiling water contains potatoes or rice this method is also super economical in fuel. Haddock can of course be bought smoked as the familiar Arbroath smokies.

Oily fish

Oily fish, such as trout, salmon, sardines, pilchards, herring, mackerel and tuna, are an especially valuable addition to our diet, despite the fact that some of them

LIKE SARDINES IN A CAN

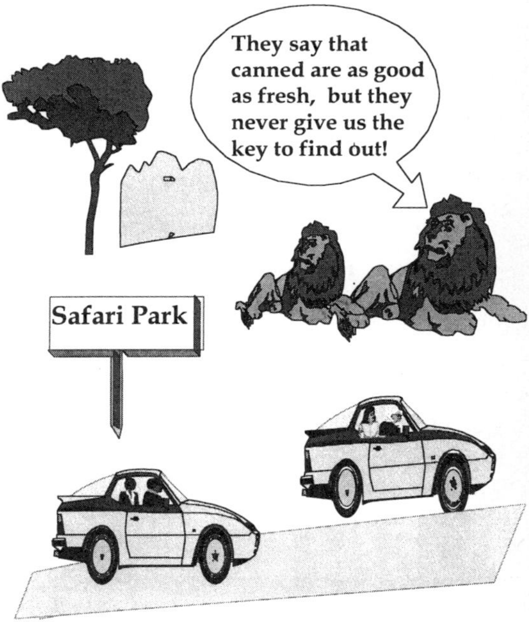

have as much fat as the same weight of red meat. Although you might think that would mean that they should be avoided, this is not the case at all, because the fat in oily fish is mostly unsaturated fat, the healthy kind.

More importantly it includes those essential fatty acids we mentioned earlier, the ones that sound like a planet in a distant solar system – the omega-3 – which help protect against heart attacks by reducing the tendency of the blood to clot and form blockages in diseased arteries.

Following a heart attack, patients are often advised by their doctor to eat oily fish to help reduce their chances of having another, and much research is currently being undertaken in an effort to work out the optimal amounts of different omega fatty acid supplements to prescribe.

Oily fish are also rich in two of the ACE vitamins, A and E, which are believed to help protect against the damage which can result in heart disease and other illnesses, as well as in the sunshine vitamin D. So even if the sun doesn't shine, we can still get our vitamin D by eating fish, as fish oil is one of the best sources.

You will have noticed that the bones of canned pilchards and salmon are always soft and chewy. Because of this, canned fish are also a useful source of calcium especially so as they also contain vitamin D which is essential for calcium to be absorbed properly from our intestines.

Fresh salmon and trout are relatively much cheaper today than they were a few years ago as a result of the development of fish farming which is now a major industry in many parts of Scotland. Most fresh salmon and trout is now farmed rather than having been caught. In the wild, numbers have been greatly depleted because of over fishing using inappropriate methods and to pollution and the blocking of the rivers which the salmon need to swim back up in order to reach their spawning grounds. Farmed salmon can be bought for a reasonable price in fishmongers although some restaurants still charge exorbitantly for it.

Kippers are herrings which have been put in brine, hung to dry and smoked for about five hours but despite this treatment are still rich in the essential fatty acids. You may wish to avoid kippers which have been artificially dyed with the browning agent FK. Personally I prefer fresh products as the smoke used to preserve bacon or fish contains some of the same nasty chemicals as cigarette smoke.

Canned fish

Canned fish is also excellent and very convenient for a quick snack. I always keep a few cans of mackerel in tangy tomato sauce in the drawer of my desk at work in case I feel peckish. Canned mackerel, sardines, pilchards and salmon have the same essential fatty acids, including the omega-3, as the fresh fish. Unfortunately, in canning tuna the natural oils are drained off, drastically reducing the omega-3s, and are replaced by vegetable oil or brine, so that its nutritional value becomes more akin to that of white fish than of oily fish.

Shellfish

Fresh shellfish are unlikely to be available in your local supermarket and you will probably have to make do with bottled or canned varieties. For the real thing we will need to abandon our trolley and nip along to the fishmonger.

Crabs and lobsters, prawns and shrimps, cockles and mussels and other shellfish are low in fat. They have a reputation for being high in cholesterol but the levels are generally no higher than in beef or poultry meat. Shrimps and lobsters are an exception with levels about half as high as those found in liver.

Cockles and mussels, especially cockles, are very rich sources of iron, and shellfish in general contain large amounts of iodine, not that we are likely to be short of iodine in Britain. At various times in history oysters and other shellfish have featured much more prominently in the British diet than they do today.

Despite their excellent nutritional qualities, shellfish have a dodgy reputation as they have sometimes been responsible for outbreaks of food poisoning. They have a nasty habit of accumulating toxins from polluted water including heavy metals and the toxins produced by certain types of algae. Blooms of these algae are becoming common in Britain and elsewhere at certain times of the year particularly where their growth is encouraged by a rich supply of nutrients in the shape of fertiliser draining off the fields and animal or human sewage.

It is important, therefore, to ensure that shellfish are purchased from a reliable source.

Fish liver oils

These are an exceptionally rich source of vitamins A and D and the omega-3 essential fatty acids and an occasional spoonful especially during winter is a good way of ensuring that we keep up our levels of vitamin D when there is too little sunshine to enable us to make very much ourselves in our skin.

Fish fingers

Most of the fish that many people, especially children, eat is in the form of fish fingers. The protein is just as good, but unfortunately, in preparing the fish fingers, saturated fat is added in the batter, depriving the fish of its healthy image. The same unfortunately applies to the fish you get from a fish and chip shop. Cast your gaze across the freezers though and you will undoubtedly hook some fish fingers which have less fat than others.

CHAPTER 12

The Dreaded Cake and Biscuit Zone

Official Recommendation: Reduce the amount of cakes and biscuits we eat by a half.

HEALTHY STARCH SPOILED WITH SUGAR, SATURATED FAT AND CHOLESTEROL

It is horrifying the amount of fat people eat in cakes and biscuits without even realising that they are eating it! It becomes all the more horrifying when the Department of Health's survey reveals that one in three adults in Britain eats biscuits every day and one in five eats cake every day.

CAKES

Take down a packet of cakes from a supermarket shelf and read the label. Don't be surprised if the cake consists of up to 50 per cent sugar; and between 15 and 30 per cent fat, as much fat as in the same weight of pork. Different types of cake vary widely in the amount of sugar and type of fat they contain but, on the average, about a third of the fat will be the harmful saturated kind, more if it's a cream cake!

Combined with the cholesterol from the eggs, all this saturated fat makes eating too much cake as bad for our arteries as daily bacon and eggs.

Digestive Biscuits

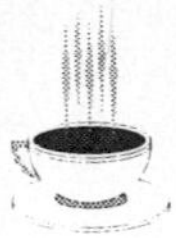

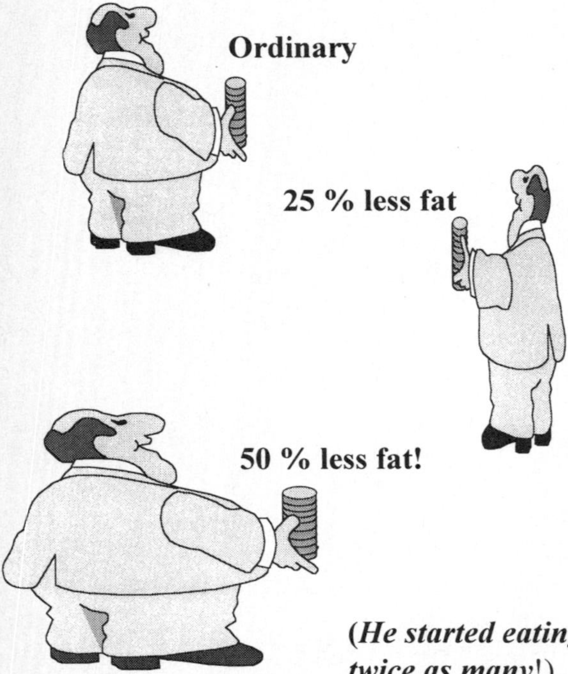

(He started eating twice as many!)

I am not suggesting we should never eat cake. It can be eaten occasionally in sensible amounts as a special treat but it is definitely not for filling up on; that is the job of high starch foods like vegetables, bread and pasta.

If the urge to buy cake becomes irresistible, all is not lost because, as always, there are lower fat options but to find out which they are we need to read the Nutrition Information on the packets and compare the fat content. In a fridge in Safeway the other day, sitting next to a box of Cadbury's Chocolate Gateau with 20 per cent fat I came across the supermarket's own Orange and Chocolate Gateau with a mere 5 per cent fat, a four-fold difference in essentially the same product! Incredibly, the Safeway product was so modest that it didn't advertise itself as low fat. We have the makings there of an interesting experiment; market the identical product in identical boxes except that one contains the words 'low fat' and see which sells the best. Is it possible that some people are such gluttons for punishment that seeing the words 'low fat' actually puts them off buying the product?

At the lower end of the fat range, jam tarts and apple pies can be a good buy. Safeway's Bramley Apple Pies for instance contain only 13 per cent fat of which little more than a quarter is the harmful saturated kind. I also came across some mince pies last Christmas in Tesco which contained 15 per cent fat overall, with less than a third of it saturated. All we have to do is Read That Label!

When we buy cakes off the display counter in a cake shop, life is not so easy because, being sold unwrapped, they are not labelled to tell us how much fat there is in them. It is always best to assume the worst and reckon that they contain as much fat as pork, a high proportion of it saturated. Most do. This is a pity because cakes that are made in small cake shop bakeries and restaurants for selling the same day, could just as well be made with a high proportion of unsaturated vegetable oil. Not that there is any need to use any significant amount of fat at all, saturated or unsaturated, when making cakes. There are lots of delicious no-fat cake recipes around.

BISCUITS

Most biscuits have even more fat than cake, and a higher proportion of it saturated. To get a feel for just how much fat biscuits contain, take down a packet of digestives from the shelf and mentally slice it into four quarters. Visualise one of those quarters as solid fat and you will get the right idea, because that is how much fat most biscuits contain, an incredible one quarter. That is one heck of a lot of fat in a product which one in three people eat every day.

Unfortunately, biscuit labels rarely state how much of the fat is saturated. In most kinds it is around half, which probably explains why the manufacturers prefer to keep quiet about it.

There is a glimmer of light on the horizon. As we cast our gaze over the biscuit shelves, our attention will almost certainly be attracted by labels which proudly proclaim that the contents have 'a quarter less fat'. Closer examination will usually reveal that even after knocking off a quarter of the fat, it still contains something like 21 per cent. Still, it is a step in the right direction. A bigger step in the right direction has been taken by Burton's who now produce the *Trim* range of biscuits with only half as much fat as the standard kind. To my taste buds their half fat digestives are even better than their high fat and they have the added advantage that they give you a breathing space in which to withdraw them from your tea before they become soggy and sink irretrievably to the bottom of the cup. Trim half fat rich tea biscuits set the standard in low fat biscuits having only 6 per cent fat overall of which less than half is the unhealthy saturated kind.

Most brands of arrowroot biscuits and Scottish oatcakes are also much better than the average biscuit. Although they typically have 20 per cent fat in total, in some brands, less than a quarter of it is saturated.

So it is now possible for a supermarket shopper to lay his or her hands on a packet of biscuits which is not too high in fat and can be eaten in moderation. But half a dozen or so brands out of the hundred or so stocked by a typical supermarket is just not good enough is it?

At the other end of the spectrum, shortbread biscuits are usually amongst the worst offenders with around 25 per cent fat, two thirds of it saturated. This is the hidden fat I keep warning about. It is the worst kind in the sense that people can go on eating large amounts of the stuff, day after day, year after year, without even realising that they are eating it.

It is good to know that by choosing carefully we can continue to enjoy the odd biscuit or two with our cup of tea. Even a nasty, higher fat biscuit is all right occasionally but, as with cake, it is important to remember that biscuits should be eaten once in a while only and definitely not be used for filling up on. As we said before – that is the job of fruit and vegetables, bread and cereals.

We don't have to *stop* eating anything! Healthy eating simply means getting the balance right, keeping down the amounts of the less healthy foods and tucking into more generous amounts of the healthy ones.

CHAPTER 13

Savoury Snacks and Sweet Temptations

Official Recommendation: Consumption should be cut by a third in adults and a half in children.

Beware the saturated fat, sugar, colourings and flavourings.

CRISPS

Crisps, like cake and biscuits, have as much fat in them as the same weight of pork. Crisps are a prime example of how to convert a healthy, first-class food, full of starch, protein and vitamins — potatoes — into junk food. Potatoes have virtually no fat, but they accumulate so much during processing that by the time they are transformed into crisps we end up with one part fat to two parts potato.

To be fair, a number of varieties of crisps are coming onto the market made with healthier, unsaturated, vegetable oil which contain very little saturated fat. If we search hard and long we may find somewhere on the supermarket shelves a brand of crisp called Highlander which is made in Scotland using sunflower oil. Highlander crisps have as much fat as ordinary crisps but only about one eighth of it is saturated.

Varieties lower in total fat are also being introduced

by most manufacturers and supermarket chains. These usually have about a third less fat than their ordinary crisps. That is still a lot of fat but it is a step in the right direction. If we must eat crisps, we should eat these and any others we can find which, like Highlander, are made using unsaturated vegetable oils and are low in saturated fat. For a few other ideas consult the Calorie and Fat Counter at the back of this book.

Most of the dozens of corn and other kinds of cheap snacks that compete for shelf space with the crisps are also over one third fat, a third of that saturated, as well as the usual additions of salt, colourings and flavourings. One crunchy snack with only a third of the fat of standard crisps, is Twiglets.

The pseudo-ethnic snacks in bigger than average packets painted to look like hessian bags, with pictures of Indian or Mexican farm labourers, offer another ray of hope despite their nauseating presentation. Although the hard-working locals depicted on the packet have certainly never tasted anything like them, some of the snacks, like Indian Popadoms, contain only half the amount of fat of crisps and almost all of it is unsaturated. The same goes for some kinds of pasta whirls. They are strong and spicy, really tasty if you like that sort of thing, again with only half fat as crisps and very little of it saturated.

Amongst the nominees for top prize for a low fat snack is the Low Fat Snack Company for their Potato Crisp Waffles. Available in the usual supermarkets, they are baked instead of fried and have only one per cent fat, not enough to bother about.

So we can still have a quick, crispy snack, so long as we Read That Label and watch what we are eating.

The trend towards bigger bags is, however, very undesirable. The 65 gram bag of lower fat crisps which replaces the typical 30g bag, may tell us that it contains *two* servings and the 100 gram bag of pizza bread may tell us that it contains *four* servings, but how many of us have the will power to put down a packet of anything until we have finished it? The healthier snack soon becomes unhealthy if we eat too much of it, and we may find ourselves in the absurd situation where we consume more fat by eating the big bag of lower fat crisps than by eating the small bag of high fat crisps.

We started off with modest 30g packets of crisps sold separately. Then they began selling them in packs of six; and now the trend is towards individual bags two or three times as big as the original. How long will it be before they start selling these in packs of six too? Is it any wonder that crisps and chocolate bars have virtually become the staple diet of so many young people?

SNACK AND CHOCOLATE BARS

It is just a short trolley dash to another of my pet hates.

A hundred different kinds of horrible sticky snack bars full of sugar and fat and coated with treacle and chocolate. Then there are those boxes of fancy chocolates. How people can stuff themselves full of this junk I shall never know!

I thought that little outburst would increase my ranking in the popularity stakes! No, I would never be so optimistic as to expect you (or myself!) and the younger members of the family to stop eating chocolate and sweets altogether, but remember they should only be eaten as a special treat and not become their staple diet.

Thankfully, many supermarkets including Tesco, Sainsbury's, Safeway and some Asda, have now, to the delight of the parents of young children, removed sweets from their checkouts, and at the time of writing a number of Safeway and Somerfield stores have taken the radical step of replacing the sweets with fresh fruit. But so much for the good news.

Unfortunately, at the same time as individual snack bars and packets of sweets are being banished from the checkouts, it is becoming increasingly difficult for parents who wish to give their children the occasional treat to buy *individual* snack bars on the main shelves. In some supermarkets all of the bars are now sold in packs of half a dozen or more. Bulk marketing of fat-laden snack bars like this makes it even more difficult for parents to limit their children's consumption of them to a sensible level and is a trend to be deplored.

For many years the best selling chocolate bar in Britain has been KitKat although it now has several strong competitors. It began life in 1935 under the name of Chocolate Crisp becoming KitKat two years later. Another old-time favourite – been to any good tea dances lately? – the Mars Bar was first sold in 1920 by the American Frank Mars. Being a very concentrated source of energy it was given to GIs as part of their rations during the Second World War. Hill climbers and mountaineers often carry a few Mars Bars with them for the same reason.

All chocolate bars are a concentrated source of energy which is very useful when our reserves are limited, but when did you last go to war or even climb a mountain? Snack bars make it all too easy to consume large numbers of calories and huge amounts of saturated fat in the blinking of an eye. KitKat is typical of most chocolate and snack bars in that about one quarter of it is fat, putting them in the same league as bacon and biscuits. A single 48g bar contains about 250 calories and 13g of fat, mostly saturated.

As can be seen from the Seek and Reduce Calorie Counter at the end of this book, a few snack bars do have

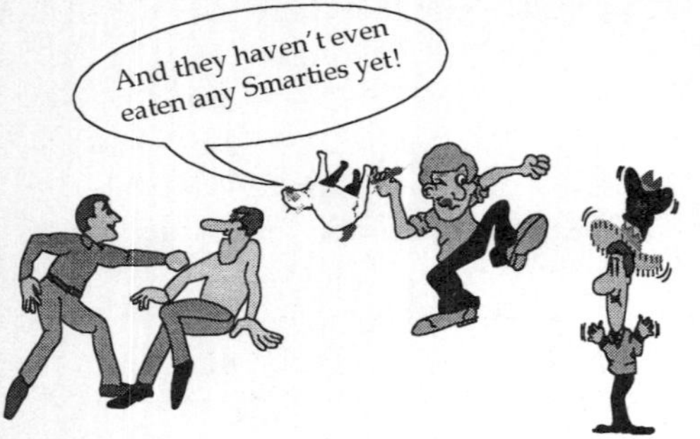

Red and Sunset Yellow, And Pink and Brilliant Blue,

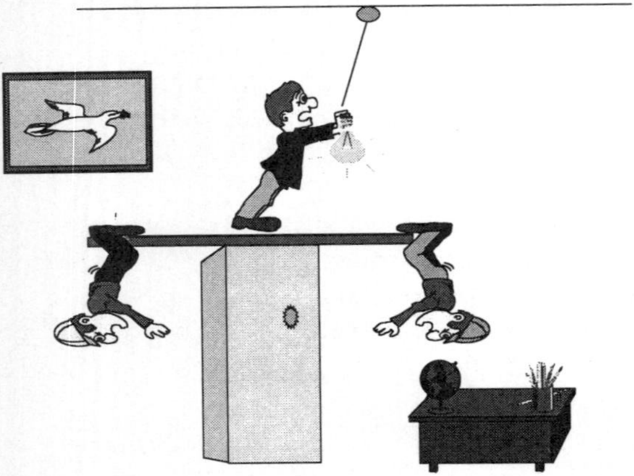

Orange and Purple and Green

significantly less fat. Mars Bars and Milky Way have a third less fat than many of their competitors. That does not, however, mean that they are low fat, as they still contain 19 and 16 per cent respectively over half of which is saturated.

Some manufacturers are still very naughty and fail to list on all of their wrappers the amount of fat. Others do so, at least on occasions, in such small print that you need a magnifying glass to read it.

If you want a snack bar that is really low in fat, try Jordan's crunchy bars. Made with oats, dried apple, honey, hazelnuts, sesame seeds, sunflower seeds and so on, they contain only about half a gram of saturated fat in each bar. Now, if we must eat sticky snacks, that is the sort we should go for.

Can I not find anything good to say about snack bars? Yes, snack bars are not entirely lacking in vitamins; they have a trace of most of the vitamins except usually vitamin C. They also have a small amount of protein.

SWEETS

Sweets, in contrast to chocolate bars, are usually entirely vitamin and protein free; pellets of tooth-rotting sugar laced with colours and flavours, and very little nutritional value apart from the energy in the sugar. But they can be tasty, and one point in their favour is that they are usually fat free.

For young children sweets are more than just something to eat. They are often used as a form of currency. 'Let me have a go with your Game Boy and I'll give you a sweet' and so on. Just as adults may buy their friends a pint or a coffee, children offer sweets. Forbidding children to eat sweets may therefore not be worth the social upheaval but their consumption should certainly not be encouraged in the home where healthier options like fresh fruit and breakfast cereals should always be readily available.

If the colourings in sweets cause you concern, go to the section on 'Additives, the good, the bad and the ugly'. Smarties boast an impressive list of artificial colourings. As well as being eaten they are often used by children as paint boxes. The colourings are as follows: titanium dioxide, to give a white colour, and carmoisine for red. Then there are sunset yellow, quinoline yellow, and brilliant blue, whose names speak for themselves. The remaining two colourings in Smarties are in fact natural substances, riboflavin (vitamin B2) to impart an orange-yellow colour, and cochineal, a red dye prepared from insects. The artificial azo dyes are often accused of causing hyperactivity in children.

It has become traditional to pick on poor old Smarties but, to be fair, most sweets have colourings of one sort or another. Chewits for example have just about as many artificial colourings as Smarties – quinoline yellow, sunset yellow, erythrosine (red) and indigo carmine (blue). Another old favourite, Rowntree's Fruit Pastilles, has its share; once more we are dazzled with sunset yellow and indigo carmine, with the red colour being created with the aid of the azo dye ponceau.

SUGAR AND TOOTH DECAY

Tooth decay as everyone knows is due to particular kinds of bacteria which live on our teeth. The plaque which gets scraped away when you visit the dental hygienist is made by the bacteria as a sort of bunker to protect themselves from bombardment by enzymes in saliva which might destroy them. Protected by the plaque, they lurk in crevices and produce acid which corrodes the teeth. They are able to make plaque more easily from sugars than from other carbohydrates like starch, and sucrose (white sugar) appears to be the best sugar of all as far as the bacteria are concerned.

What the bacteria like best is a constant supply of sugar, so consuming one sweet snack after another or prolonged sucking of sweets without cleaning the teeth in between is ideal for them. Children should be encouraged to eat sweet things only occasionally and to clean their teeth afterwards to avoid the build up of plaque. Tooth decay starts very early in life. A recent nation-wide survey of young children carried out by the British Association for the Study of Community Dentistry showed that in the West of Scotland where the water did not have added fluoride, children as young as five years had on the average three decayed or filled teeth. At that rate virtually all of their teeth would be likely to suffer decay by their early teens. Top marks went to children in Bromsgrove, Redditch and Solihull where the average was one filling for every two children.

ON YOUR WAY TO BED AT NIGHT BRUSH YOUR TEETH SHINING BRIGHT

Around the corner from the sweet counter you will come across a shelf full of toothbrushes and toothpaste for this very purpose. Despite the introduction of fluoride toothpaste and the addition of one part per million fluoride to water supplies in many areas, tooth decay is still a major problem. Fluoride helps to strengthen growing teeth but will not provide complete protection against decay and if we live in a fluoridated area it should not be seen as an excuse for poor dental hygiene. It certainly does not absolve us from the need to cut down on the sugary snacks and keep our teeth clean.

Here is a thought to ponder. You probably drink tea or coffee, so if the water supply in the area where you live has fluoride added you will get a daily dose. Children on the other hand rarely drink tea or coffee, either they don't like it or, as it is a stimulant, we prefer not to encourage them to drink it. Moreover, few children drink water directly from the tap. Most of what they drink comes in bottles, but from where? You may live in an area where the water contains added fluoride, but what if the lemonade and fruit juice drinks your children use to quench their thirst with are produced in a part of the country where the water does not have added fluoride? Apart from the small volume of water remaining with boiled vegetables, they will gain very little of the benefit of the local fluoridation.

In reality, as most water supplies now have fluoride added, the reverse is more likely to be the case. Even if fluoride is not added to your water supply, it could well be present in most of the water your children drink. This creates a dilemma for parents who are opposed to the addition of fluoride to water supplies, while at the same time providing an opportunity for those who are in favour but live in an area where it isn't added. If you are concerned one way or the other, just look at the label, find out the address of the company that produces it, give them a ring and ask if their water is fluoridated. The problem is that the sugar and carbonic acid in most fizzy drinks probably does as much harm to teeth as the fluoride does good.

If, as is preferable, the family's favourite drink is *pure* fruit juice it is not going to be easy to find out whether the soils of the plantation in South Africa or the USA or wherever the fruit was grown contain fluoride, so don't worry in that case, just use fluoride toothpaste.

SUGAR: DON'T LET IT DISTORT YOUR DIET

It is not only sweets that contain sugar. It is added in quite unnecessarily large amounts to all sorts of things,

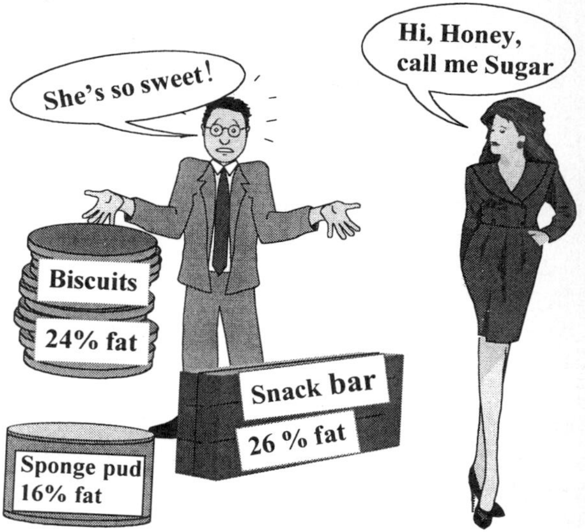
She's so sweet!
Hi, Honey, call me Sugar
Biscuits
24% fat
Snack bar
26 % fat
Sponge pud
16% fat

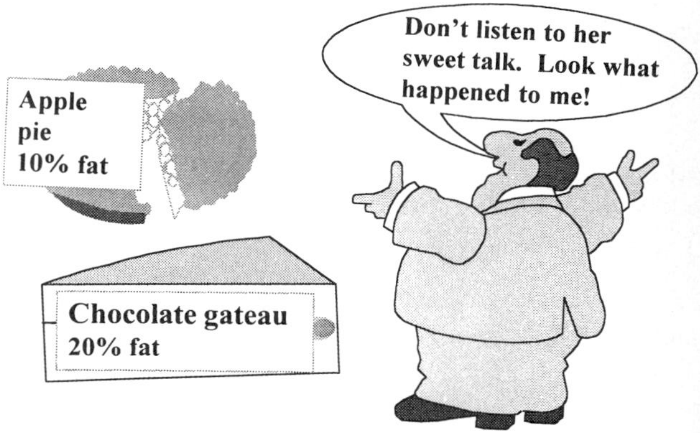
Don't listen to her sweet talk. Look what happened to me!
Apple pie 10% fat
Chocolate gateau 20% fat

like cakes and biscuits, sticky puddings and those chocolate bars, even some breakfast cereals.

Sugar is perfectly acceptable in sensible amounts. Many healthy foods, like fresh fruit, contain a lot of sugar. It is not quite the same as the white sugar you buy by the kilogram in bags, but even the odd spoonful of white sugar in your tea won't do you any harm. The problem is that ridiculous amounts of sugar are added to some foods and drinks. Unlike the cup of tea with its single spoonful, a can of Coke and similar fizzy drinks contain about seven spoonfuls of sugar. Many children's breakfast cereals like Frosties and Sugar Puffs are plastered with sugar. There is a huge amount in most cakes and biscuits and sticky puddings. Sugar, as we have seen, is even added to baked beans.

The table below shows the amount of sugar in some common snacks. In the fruit and pure fruit juice all of the sugar is part of the fruit and none will have been added whereas at the other extreme, in the fizzy drinks all of the sugar has been added. This table is Just for Fun. I am not suggesting you should always choose your food according to how much sugar it contains. The amount of fat and total calories are much more important considerations.

HOW MANY TEASPOONS?

		Number of teaspoons of sugar (1 tsp = 5g)
Snacks		
Mars Bar	bar (100g)	13
Boiled sweets	100g	17
Chocolate digestive biscuits	4 biscuits	4
Cake	slice (100g)	8

Drinks		
Coca Cola	one 330 ml can	7
Pure orange juice	a large 330ml mug	7
Cup of tea		1 or less
Breakfast cereals	one bowl (50g)	
Sugar Puffs		5
Rice Krispies		1
Frosties		4
Cornflakes		1
Baked Beans	one small can (205g)	2.5
Canned fruit	one bowl (105g)	
Fruit cocktail in juice		1.5
Fruit cocktail in syrup		3
Fresh fruit	medium without skin	
Banana	(100g)	4
Orange	(160g)	2.5
Apple	(100g)	2.5

It makes sense to avoid foods and drinks which are obviously excessively sweet, but having said that, sweet things are all right for a special treat from time to time, and I would never stop eating baked beans just because they contain sugar, as they are so nutritious otherwise.

Avoid being tricked by the sweet taste of added sugar into eating foods which also contain a lot of unhealthy saturated fat.

Sugar is a temptress who, with her overpowering appeal to the taste buds, can seduce us into eating all kinds of unhealthy, highly processed, high-fat, low-vitamin foods, to which she has been added, such as cakes, biscuits and snack bars.

Better by far to satisfy our sweet tooth by tucking into lots of apples and pears, bananas, grapes and strawberries and the other delights of the fresh fruit section which provide us with vitamins, minerals and fibre as well as sugar, without inflicting upon us unwanted saturated fat and additives.

ARTIFICIAL SWEETENERS

Artificial sweeteners are for people who need or wish to reduce their consumption of sugars but cannot give up their liking for sweetness even if the sweetness tastes very different from the sweetness of sugar. Manufacturers like sugar substitutes because they are cheaper, mainly because much smaller amounts are required. Saccharin, for example, is 300 times sweeter than sugar, so only one three hundredth as much is needed, reducing transport and handling costs if nothing else. The other two most commonly used sweeteners are about 200 times sweeter than sugar. The problem is that artificial sweeteners are added automatically to almost every diet and low calorie product on the market to replace the sweetness of the sugar that has been removed. As the range of products to which they are added increases, they are being rammed in increasing amounts down the throats of those of us who can do perfectly well without either sugar or artificial sweeteners.

As they are added to more and more products, the question of safety becomes more urgent. Saccharin has been around for over 100 years, but we are still not certain whether it is absolutely safe. Those suspicious of it point to the experiments which show that in enormous doses it can cause cancer in rats but people who consume more saccharin than the average have not been shown to be more likely to get cancer. It is added to many soft drinks, canned foods, ice lollies, confectionery and so on.

Another popular sweetener is acesulfame-K which turns up in products as diverse as low calorie yoghurts and baked beans. It is about 200 times sweeter than sugar. It is more resistant to heat than saccharin and so can be used for products which undergo cooking.

Aspartame is about 180 times sweeter than sugar. It was first introduced into Britain in the mid-Eighties. It loses its sweetness on contact with heat and so is not suitable for cooking. It is made from two amino acids which, as you know, are the building blocks of proteins, called aspartic acid and phenylalanine. Because it contains phenylalanine it should be avoided by the one child in 16,000 who suffers from the rare genetic condition known as phenylketonuria, and who is unable to deal with this amino acid and become ill if they consume too much of it. Aspartame turns up in a wide variety of diet soft drinks and low calorie foods. Sold under the name of NutraSweet or Canderel it is also available in sachets for sweetening tea or coffee, to which it imparts its own unique taste. The recent Health Survey for England found that only half of the men and one in three of the women interviewed added sugar to their tea, many of the remainder presumably using artificial sweeteners.

Is there a limit to how much of the artificial sweeteners we can safely consume and, if so, what is the limit? There is an organisation called the Committee on Toxicity which looks at additives like sweeteners and decides whether to set what they call an Acceptable Daily Intake, abbreviated as ADI. So how do they decide what is an acceptable daily intake? The way they do it is to find out the maximum amount which can be added to an animal's diet without causing an adverse effect, and divide it by 100. It is very crude but as you can't carry out experiments on people, feeding them increasing doses until they keel over, that is about the best they can do.

The acceptable daily intake for a 60kg adult is 300mg of saccharin; 540mg of acesulfame and 2,400mg of aspartame. For a child weighing half as much, reduce these amounts by a half.

This information is about as useful as knowing how many times the annual banana crop if laid end to end would encircle the world, the reason being that we haven't a clue as to how much artificial sweetener we are consuming. If a product contains a sweetener it must be stated on the label but the manufacturer is not obliged to say how much of it there is, and virtually never does.

Manufacturers have this perverse notion that if they don't add sugar to their products they must add artificial sweeteners instead. Artificial sweeteners do nothing worth while. They don't kill bacteria or moulds, they don't prevent food from going rancid. All they do is give it a peculiar kind of sickly sweetness and encourage the sweet tooth. I for one don't want artificial sweeteners added to my 'healthy' baked beans or low fat rice pudding any more than I want sugar. So manufacturers of diet products read my lips. W-E D-O-N-'T W-A-N-T T-H-E S-U-G-A-R I-N R-E-D-U-C-E-D S-U-G-A-R P-R-O-D-U-C-T-S A-U-T-O-M-A-T-I-C-A-L-L-Y R-E-P-L-A-C-E-D B-Y A-R-T-I-F-I-C-I-A-L S-W-E-E-T-E-N-E-R-S. .

CHOOSING THE HEALTHY OFFICE SNACK

For a low fat, low calorie snack choose an apple or banana, perhaps with a slice of bread, or a yoghurt and leave the crisps, biscuits and chocolate bars alone. The table below compares the calories in a few familiar snacks.

	Size	Kcal in each portion	Fat in each portion
Solid snacks			
High calorie			
KitKat	48g bar	240	12.5
Mars Bar	65g bar	294	11.4
Standard digestive biscuits	4 biscuits	283	13
Ordinary crisps	30g bag	164	11
Lower calorie			
Potato Crisp Waffles	30g bag	99	Trace
Wholemeal bread	1 slice	72	0.8
Trim rich tea biscuits	4 biscuits	122	4.2
Apple	100g	42	Trace
Banana	160g	93	Trace
Very low fat natural yoghurt	120g pot	60	Trace
Drinks			
Semi-skimmed milk	250ml glass	122	4.2
Pure orange juice	250ml glass	113	Nil
Lucozade	330ml can	248	Nil
Coke	330ml can	142	Nil
Diet Coke	330ml can	1	Nil
Mug of tea with 15mls semi-skimmed milk and one teaspoon (5g) of sugar		27	Trace

If you want an energy rich drink with natural sugar and extra nutrients, drink semi-skimmed milk or pure fruit juice. If weight control is the main aim, tea, even with a spoonful of sugar, and the diet varieties of fizzy drinks may be for you, but take the more nutritious drinks from time to time as well.

CHAPTER 14

Drinks: Fizzy, Hot and Intoxicating

THE COLA ZONE – CANS OF LOTS OF ADDITIVES

Most supermarkets stock around 50 different kinds of fizzy drinks and basically all most of them contain is sugar, colourings and flavourings, dissolved in carbonated water. Many of the diet varieties don't even contain the sugar, which is replaced by artificial sweeteners, and so are of no nutritional value whatsoever. We may as well just drink tap water. It's a lot cheaper. That said, a lot of people like the taste of fizzy drinks, and who doesn't enjoy the odd can of Coke or IrnBru from time to time, so is there any harm in them? It depends on whether we regard what we drink as an integral part of our diet, or just as an alternative to water to quench our thirst. So long as the colourings, flavourings and artificial sweeteners are not doing us any harm, then the diet varieties may be perfectly acceptable for those of us who are certain we are getting enough energy and vitamins from the food we eat and just want a pleasant way of quenching our thirst.

At the other extreme, the main contender for the most 'fattening' fizzy drink is Lucozade with no less than 18 per cent sugar (mostly glucose). But as it is marketed as a source of energy for those not up to taking solid food and as an energy booster for athletes, the sugar content is perfectly acceptable. Despite this traditional image, even some Lucozade varieties are now available light with only half the usual amount of sugar.

For myself though, I always look upon drinks as a nutritional opportunity, homing in on the vitamins and carbohydrate in the pure fruit juices and ignoring for the most part the fizzy varieties. Pure fruit juice contains about 10 per cent natural sugar. For people who need a fair amount of energy but may have small appetites, like children and the elderly, this natural sugar is a welcome, easily consumed source of energy. If we want to wean our children off sugary/high fat snack bars and fatty crisps, but are afraid that in the process we may deprive them of valuable calories, pure fruit juice is the answer. It provides a rapid means of replacing the lost energy, with the added bonus of a daily shot of vitamin C.

Although pure fruit juice is the healthy shopper's drink of choice, obtaining energy from the white sugar in the non-diet varieties of fizzy drinks is no worse than obtaining it from the saturated fat in snack bars and crisps. The odd can of fizzy drink *instead* of a snack bar or packet of crisps is not going to do us any harm, so long as we remember that nutritionally pure fruit juice is so much better and is the drink to include in our staple diet. Ironically, owing to the mild laxative effect of pure fruit juice – normally a big extra point in its favour – if you suffer the misfortune of contracting gastro-enteritis with severe diarrhoea, a fizzy drink like 7-UP which contains sugar but no fruit juice is a better bet, after getting rid of the fizz, for replacing lost fluids.

Why should not *pure* fruit juice be given a fizz for people who like their drinks fizzy? Fizzy grape juice is, in fact, available in most supermarkets alongside the big cartons of pure juice in what look at first glance like wine bottles. It is a bit more expensive than the non-fizzy varieties, but is still a good everyday buy as well as being an excellent soft drink for parties and receptions. Not that money is any object for fizzy drink fanatics. How many people do you see buying their Cola or 7-UP or whatever in expensive cans when they could buy the identical product in two-litre plastic bottles for a half of the cost per litre?

SQUASHES FOR DILUTING

While on the subject of fruit juices, what about the bottles of concentrated fruit juices for diluting with water? Some of these such as Ribena Blackcurrant Juice and Robinson's Lemon Barley have been around for generations. Many of them are regarded as good, healthy drinks particularly by middle-aged people who were encouraged to drink them as children. They were indeed one of the few reliable, year round sources of vitamin C before pure fruit juice became so readily available. They also had the advantage that because they were highly concentrated and contained preservatives, they would keep for a long time after being opened, without the need for a refrigerator.

Even though nearly every home now has a fridge, squashes may still be tempting to those of us who have a long walk home or to the bus stop with our shopping as one bottle of concentrate to be diluted one in four with water when we get home is a lot easier to carry than five cartons of pure juice already at drinking strength. Unlike pure fruit juices, squashes tend to have colours and flavours, artificial sweeteners and preservatives added to them. The better quality products like Ribena and Robinson's concentrated juices tend to use natural flavourings and colourings like grape skin extracts and beta-carotene, but they still need the preservatives and, in the latter case, artificial sweeteners.

For supermarket shoppers without a car, it can be well worth investing in a taxi home from time to time to stock up on the heavy, long lasting items like pure fruit juice and potatoes, unless you are blessed with a local supermarket like ours which, after you have selected your shopping, will put it into boxes and, for a modest charge, deliver it to your home. Most of the larger supermarkets now have their own taxi ranks, with taxis for the asking, while nearly all in-town and small supermarkets have a telephone where you can call for a taxi.

Nutritionally, the best drink of all is semi-skimmed or skimmed milk. As we saw when we were at the dairy counter, it is a source of first-class protein, carbohydrate, calcium and vitamins. Children who refuse to drink pure milk may be persuaded to drink it in the form of milk shakes, choosing those varieties made from skimmed and semi-skimmed milk with natural colourings and flavourings.

HOT DRINKS

Although not so abundant as fizzy drinks, there is still a big enough selection of hot drinks to make the choice interesting. To begin with there are the ubiquitous teas and coffees, of which there are always dozens of blends to choose from. Nutritionally, neither tea nor coffee are of much value until (semi-skimmed) milk and sugar are added to provide some protein and carbohydrate. The exception to this is that tea is generally regarded as a good source of fluoride, which may help strengthen the teeth of those of us living in areas where the drinking water does not have fluoride added. Not all teas will contain the same amount of fluoride, the actual amounts present depending on the variety and whether it was grown in a part of the world where the soil is rich in fluoride.

If you have young children in, or visiting, the house always buy tea bags rather than loose tea and make individual cups rather than huge pots. Before the days of tea bags, hundreds of children used to get badly scalded each year as a result of grabbing the ends of tablecloths and pulling pots of boiling tea over themselves. Now that tea bags encourage us to make our tea in individual mugs, the volume of tea children get over them is much smaller and, as it doesn't stay hot in a mug so long as in a pot, it is less likely to cause serious harm. Not many doctors can claim to have prevented so much suffering as the inventor of the tea bag!

In most countries it is the custom to drink tea neat and to savour, as one would wine, the delicate aromas of the different varieties before swallowing them, but tea drinkers in Britain usually commit the ultimate sin of destroying its subtle flavours by adding milk and sugar, the same people no doubt who are prepared to add water to a delicate Scotch malt whisky! I should talk! The only way I can stand the taste of whisky is to add a spoonful to a cup of tea (Gaelic whisky) and there is no way I can drink tea without adding milk to it!

According to the recent Department of Health's survey of our eating habits, only about one in two men and one in three women now add sugar to their tea, some doing without, the rest using artificial sweeteners. Is banishing sugar from tea an effective means of weight control? If we find that a single spoonful of sugar adds enough sweetness to our cup (personally I'm down to half a teaspoonful), it is hardly worth bothering with artificial sweeteners as a spoonful (5g) only provides about 20kcals, so seven cups a day would only add up to 140kcals, less than the calories in two ordinary digestive biscuits.

Fizzy drink enthusiasts have much more of a problem

as a can of ordinary Coke for example has the equivalent of seven spoonfuls of sugar, so we needn't feel too guilty about the single spoonful of sugar in our tea. The amount of milk people add to their tea varies enormously so it is difficult to generalise as to how many extra kcals are added in the milk, especially as it depends on whether the milk is full fat, semi-skimmed or skimmed. The amount of semi-skimmed milk in the plastic pots provided in restaurants (15ml) would provide a modest extra 7kcals.

Coffee is also low in nutrients, apart from the vitamin niacin, and is drunk for its stimulatory rather than nutritional content.

As well as tea and coffee the adjacent shelves provide a choice of what are often regarded as bedtime drinks, like Build-up powder, Complan, Horlicks and Ovaltine. An advantage of these over coffee or tea is that they are fortified with vitamins A, D and B12. As these vitamins do not occur naturally in cereal grains, fruit and vegetable foods, they are a good drink throughout the day for vegetarians and others who eat very little animal food. As a bedtime drink they are preferable to tea and coffee or cocoa in that they do not contain stimulants to keep us awake.

ALCOHOLIC DRINKS

Although not generally thought of as such, alcoholic drinks are indeed a food, albeit of a very limited kind. They have no protein to speak of and are lacking in most vitamins but they certainly contain an abundance of calories, from the unfermented sugar and starch as well as from the alcohol itself. It may come as a surprise to learn that alcohol contains even more calories than the same weight of white sugar and almost as much as fat.

The average daily consumption of alcohol in the UK is

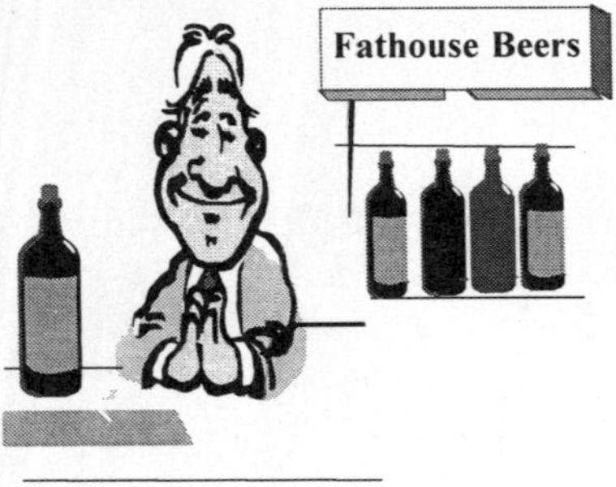
Fathouse Beers

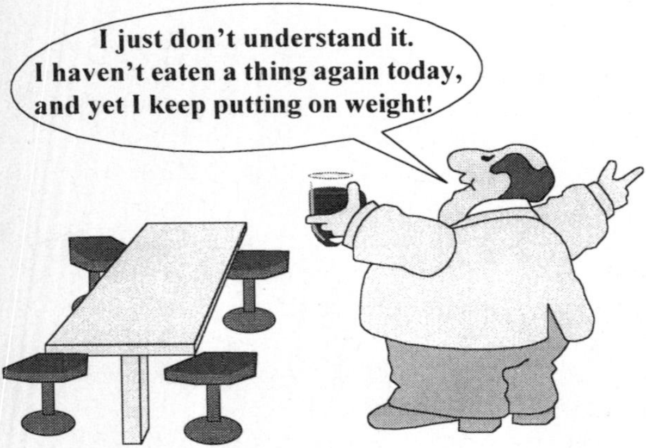
I just don't understand it.
I haven't eaten a thing again today,
and yet I keep putting on weight!

around 20gm, or two and a half units. A unit is 8gm of alcohol and is equivalent to half a pint of ordinary strength beer or lager or a small glass of wine. A lot of people drink much more than this of course while many drink none at all. This amount of alcohol alone excluding the carbohydrate, provides about 140kcal.

So that's why beer drinkers get fat bellies, is it?

You're right, going down to the pub several nights a week and downing a few pints or sitting in front of the telly with half a dozen cans is as fattening as stuffing yourself full of cream cakes. But seriously, just how fattening are alcoholic drinks? A typical can (440ml) of beer or lager has around 135kcal, as much as a Bird's Eye Dairy Cream Eclair! Drink half a dozen and that's a massive 800kcal. Extra strength lagers have over twice as many calories per can.

Unfortunately cans of beer or bottles of any other alcoholic drink for that matter, rarely state exactly how many calories they contain. An exception to the rule are cans of no or low alcohol beers and lagers which do sometimes reveal their calorie count. It is very much in their interests to do so, to tap into the weight watching as well as the breathalyser watching market. The label on a can of Tennent's LA reveals an alcohol content of 80kcal which is typical of low alcohol lagers and little more than half that of ordinary lagers. You can get lower. Barbican for instance has about a third less calories than the average low alcohol lager.

Cider tends to have slightly more calories per pint than beer or lager.

Wine has more than twice as many calories as the same volume of beer but as we tend to drink smaller volumes that is not so bad as it seems. A glass of medium wine gives us about 105kcal, assuming we drink our supermarket bottles of wine at home in wine glasses

(140ml) and not by the coffee mug! It naturally varies a bit according to the wine, a dry white wine for instance having about a third fewer calories than a sweet white wine.

Fortified wines in turn have twice as many calories as the same volume of ordinary wine, but again reducing the size of our glass by over a half to the pub measure of 50ml prevents the number of calories from increasing.

Whisky, gin and other spirits have nearly twice as many calories as the fortified wine, while liqueurs have even more calories than the same glass filled with fresh single cream. Fortunately the pub measures are small but what about the amounts drunk at home?

THE BOOZER'S CALORIE COUNTER

	Kcal/100ml (average)	**Size of typical can or glass**	**Kcal/can or glass**
Beers and lagers	31	440 ml can	135
Barbican low alcohol lager	*12*	*440 ml can*	*55*
Cider	40	440 ml can	175
Wine	75	140 ml glass	105
Low alcohol wine	*25*	*140 ml glass*	*35*
Fortified wines	125	50 ml glass	65
Spirits	200	25 ml glass	50
Liqueurs	300	25 ml glass	75

Should alcoholic drinks be universally condemned or do they have a part in a book on healthy eating? Until recently, they stood accused, tried and convicted but then a number of research studies were published which seemed to suggest that a moderate intake of alcohol, like a glass of wine at a meal, helped to protect against heart attacks. The problem is that most people in Britain do not drink a glass of wine as part of a healthy Mediterranean type meal with fish and fresh fruit and vegetables but are more likely to consume several pints of beer or lager in the pub as an adjunct to pie and chips. The greatest reduction in heart disease will come from an improvement in overall diet and an increase in exercise levels, not a daily alcohol fix. An evening at the local leisure centre will have greater health benefits than one spent at the pub.

CHAPTER 15

Read That Label!

Food labels can provide us with a great deal of information about the food we are buying, substituting to some extent for the sense of smell and touch we use when buying fresh fruit and vegetables.

DESCRIBING THE PRODUCT

Strawberry flavour but no strawberries

The law says that the name of a product should not be misleading, but names will be misleading unless we understand the words and expressions used by manufacturers to describe their products. Take for example the use of the word 'flavour'. When this appears in the name of a product, like 'strawberry flavour yoghurt' it usually means that the product contains a mixture of chemicals resembling the flavour of strawberries but no actual strawberries. There is no law which states that cheese and onion flavoured crisps need contain any cheese or onion, or strawberry flavoured yoghurt any strawberries. If, however, we see a product described as 'strawberry yoghurt' then it must contain strawberries. It is the use of the magic word 'flavour' which makes all the difference, enabling the real fruit to disappear at a wave of the manufacturer's wand. Including 'flavour' in the description completely absolves the manufacturer from using the real thing.

Every picture tells a story

If the yoghurt has a picture of strawberries on the pot that is a sign that it does indeed contain strawberries, because pictures are not allowed to mislead and a yoghurt which derives its strawberry flavour from artificial flavourings rather than from strawberries is not permitted to show a picture of strawberries on the pot. Having said that it doesn't mean that there are necessarily very many strawberries added.

The name of a product should also tell us if the food has undergone any type of process. Typical examples are smoked herring, dried apricots, UHT milk.

Low fat and reduced sugar: lower than what?

Beware of wrappers which advertise a product as 'low fat', as there is currently no law to say how low 'low' has to be. There are, however, voluntary guidelines for manufacturers to follow if they make such a claim. A 'low fat' product should have no more than 5 per cent by weight of fat.

'Reduced fat' is another expression to watch out for. A 'reduced fat' product should have no more than three quarters of the fat of the regular product.

Other wording such as 'lower fat' can mean anything. Comparative claims will in any case always mean different things depending on what kind of food we are talking about. For instance, a reduced fat margarine may contain only half as much fat as a comparable margarine, but still have ten times more than a reduced fat rice pudding, simply because there was so much more fat in the margarine to begin with.

Sugar claims should also be viewed with caution. Some manufacturers may put 'reduced sugar' on their product because it has less sugar than their own standard product, but not necessarily less sugar that the standard product of another manufacturer. The only way to find out which is the best buy is to check out the nutritional information on the label.

Low and reduced calorie: compared with what?
Many products claim that they are 'low calorie'. Does this have any more meaning than 'low fat'? Surprisingly it does. Manufacturers are only allowed to describe a product as 'low calorie' if it has no more than 40kcal in every 100g (3.5oz) – about the same as a very low fat yoghurt.

The expression 'reduced calorie' is a bit more ambiguous. It can be used if the product contains less than 75 per cent of the calories of comparable products. But we must beware of being lulled into a false sense of security by reduced calorie claims so that we eat more of a product than we otherwise would, otherwise we may end up consuming more calories, not less. The same applies to reduced fat products. Don't use the low fat tag as an excuse for eating more!

Throwing light on 'Lite'
Another common expression which pops up with increasing regularity all over the supermarket, from the margarine to the biscuit counter, is 'light' or 'lite'. It too can mean almost anything. Firstly, what is the product lighter in? Seeing 'light' written on, say, a packet of digestive biscuits a slimmer might well assume that they are lower in calories than standard biscuits and buy them, but if we read the Nutrition Information on the labels we may well find that they are lower in fat – which is good – but just as high in calories.

If a product is described as 'lite' it should mean that it is lighter in fat or calories than a comparable product but this does not necessarily mean that it is a healthy low fat food. After all, a 'light margarine' may be commendably lower in fat than ordinary margarine, but it will still be very high in fat compared to a 'light yoghurt' which will have hardly any fat at all. For example Flora Extra Light margarine has 39 per cent compared with Asda Very Low Fat, Light Yoghurt which has virtually no fat (0.1g).

Read That Label!

Pringles Original Potato Chips

NUTRITION INFORMATION, AVERAGE PER:/NAHRWERTE PRO:/ INFORMACION NUTRIMENTAL POR 100G:/INFORMATION NUTRITIONNELLE POUR:/ GEMIDDELDE VOEDINGSWAARDE PER:

ENERGY/ ENERGIE/CONTENIDO ENERGETICO / VALEUR ENERGETIQUE / ENERGETISCHE WAARDE	570KCAL,
PROTEIN / EIWEISS / PROTEINAS. / PROTEINES / EIWITTEN	5.9 G
CARBOHYDRATE / KOHLENHYDRATE / CARBOHIDRATOS. / GLUCIDES / KOOLHYDRATEN	51 G
OF WHICH SUGARS / DAVON ZUCKER / AZUCARES.. / DONT SUCRES / WAARVAN SUIKERS	0.8 G
FAT / FETT / GRASAS. / LIPIDES / VETTEN	38 G
OF WHICH SATURATES / DAVON GESATTIGT / GRASA SATURADA. / DONT SATURES / WAARVAN VERZADIGO	9.9 G
FIBRE / BALASTSTOFFE / FIBRA DIETETICA / FIBRES ALIMENTAIRES / VOEDINGSVEZELS	3.0 G
SODIUM / NATRIUM / SODIO / SODIUM / NATRIUM	0.6 G

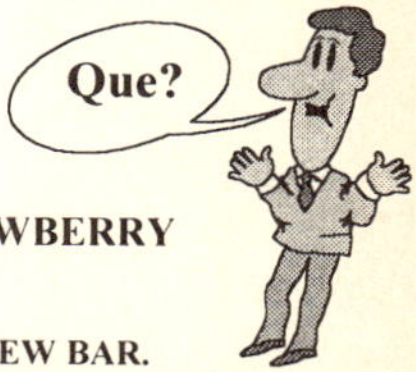

MATLOW'S GIANT STRAWBERRY REFRESHERS

STRAWBERRY FLAVOUR CHEW BAR.

Ingredients: Glucose Syrup, Sugar, Vegetable Oil, Gelling Agent Gelatine, Tartaric Acid, Emulsifier Glycerol Monostearate, Citric Acid Flavourings, Colours E104, E110, E124, E132, E150.

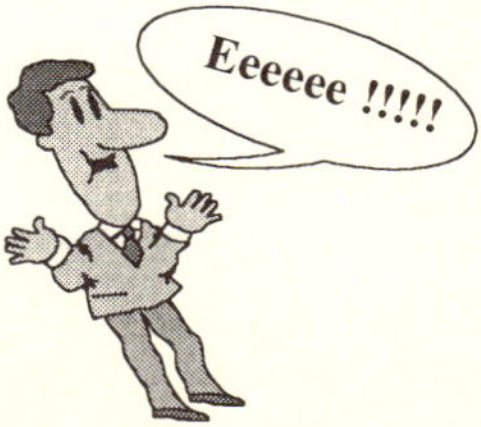

THE LIST OF INGREDIENTS

Packaged foods must by law carry a list of ingredients which have to be listed in descending order of weight. Therefore if the list on the side of a carton of a fruit juice drink reads: 'water, sugar, fruit juice, natural flavours', this means that the drink consists mainly of water, followed by sugar, with fruit juice in third place, while the flavourings which are needed in only minute amounts are listed last.

RULES ABOUT ADDITIVES

The additives present in the food should be stated in the list of ingredients together with their function. If for example potassium sorbate is added as a preservative it should be written on the label as 'preservative – potassium sorbate' or if saccharin is added as an artificial sweetener it should be stated thus: 'artificial sweeteners – saccharin'.

This enables us to avoid additives we are not happy about and is especially important to people who have allergies to particular additives like the azo dyes used as colourings. Manufacturers can provide either the full name of the additive or its E number. We will learn how to decipher the infamous E numbers later.

NUTRITIONAL INFORMATION

Almost all manufacturers now include on the label a Nutrition Information Table in anticipation of its becoming a legal requirement. All of the tables contain four basic pieces of information. The first and most vital for the weight watcher is the number of calories in each 100g (3.5oz) portion. The figure is nearly always given in both kJ and kcal. Ignore the kJ figure, as in Britain everyone measures their calories in kcals.

Of more importance than the number of calories is the

amount of fat, as fat, particularly saturated fat, is something we all need to avoid consuming too much of, even if we are trying to put on, rather than lose, weight. What we need to know most is what proportion of the fat is the undesirable saturated kind, but not all manufacturers yet reveal this.

The amount of protein and carbohydrate is expressed as grams per 100 grams of product. Some manufacturers also reveal how much of the carbohydrate is sugar. In many products most of the sugar is added white sugar but it has to be remembered that fruit and some vegetables like sweetcorn contain a lot of sugar of their own. Manufacturers are not obliged to state in their Nutrition Information Table how much sugar they have added to their product to tempt the sweet toothed to buy it, but we have a way of making them talk! Remember the obligatory list of ingredients where each ingredient has to be listed by descending order of weight? If, for example, in a fruit juice drink, sugar features higher up the list than fruit juice, you then know that the drink contains more sugar than fruit juice.

The amount of each constituent is given in the Nutrition Information Table as grams per 100 grams of product (including the weight of the water) regardless of the size of the can or packet. This enables us to compare one product with another. You may find it easier to visualise these figures as a percentage – 25g fat per 100g meaning that the product is 25 per cent fat. If the product is a liquid its fat content is given as grams per 100mls, which is much the same as grams per 100 grams, as a ml conveniently weighs about a gram. As well as the amount in 100 grams, some labels also tell us how much protein, carbohydrate and so on there is in a typical serving, or in the actual bar of chocolate or packet of crisps etc, if it weighs less than 100 grams.

You may have wondered what the big **e** stands for which follows the weight of the product. This means that the weight given is the *average* quantity in the pack or can, but the weight of individual packs may vary slightly from the average.

Knowing how much salt has been added to processed food is especially important for people who need to watch their blood pressure so that they can compare different brands to find the ones with the lowest amount, and the provision of this information has recently become a legal requirement. A high fibre content is also a good selling point, and the amount of fibre is now included on most cans of peas and beans to remind us that they have almost as much fibre as the same amount of high fibre breakfast cereals. Manufacturers are, however, only obliged to provide this information if they make a claim like 'high fibre' or 'low sugar' for their product. Having made such a claim they must then back it up by revealing on the label just how much fibre or sugar it contains so that the shopper can decide for him or herself if the claim is really justified.

Not many companies yet provide a list of the main vitamins and minerals in their products unless, like breakfast cereals, they have been artificially fortified with them. This is surprising as it could be very much in their interest to do so boosting sales amongst shoppers on the look out for particular nutrients. For example, Bird's Eye, on the packet of their Boil in the Bag Liver and Onion meal while providing the basic calorie, protein, fat and carbohydrate information in their standard nutrition table, fail to reveal that their product is one of the richest sources of vitamin B12, vitamin A, and readily absorbable iron around.

FOOD THAT DOES NOT CONTAIN ANY NUTRITIONAL INFORMATION

Food that is sold unwrapped (such as freshly baked bread and cakes, meat and sweets) does not have to carry a list of ingredients. In theory a notice nearby should give some information about the product including the main additives it contains, but in practice such information is often lacking. Surprisingly, although bottles of fruit juice and squash carry a list of ingredients, bottles and cans of beer, lager and wine and spirits do not, even though they frequently contain preservatives and colourings. Some lagers and ciders, for instance, contain the yellow dye tartrazine to which some people are allergic, while others are coloured with caramel. Low alcohol beers and lagers may reveal the number of calories they contain, but that is about all they give away. The implementation of proposals for the improved labelling of alcoholic drinks is long overdue.

AVOIDING FOOD POISONING, DATE MARKS

'Use before'

Labels also provide a vital piece of information which helps us to avoid food poisoning, namely the 'use by' date. A 'use by' date is given on highly perishable foods such as meat and dairy products and ready prepared meals on which bacteria could grow and give us a nasty stomach ache. We should always store the food according to the manufacturer's instructions and make sure that the food is eaten by this date. It is illegal to sell food after its 'use by' date. If the label says that the product should be kept in the fridge at 1-5 °C and gives 5 June as the 'use by' date, if we don't have a fridge we will have to eat it earlier otherwise it might have gone off by the 5th.

'Best before'

Most foods which can safely be kept for a longish period like biscuits carry a 'best before' date. Once this date has passed it doesn't mean that the food is necessarily dangerous but it may be passed its best, the biscuits for example may not be as crisp as they were.

STORAGE INSTRUCTIONS

Storage instructions have to be clearly provided on the labels of perishable products and these should obviously be followed. If it says the product should be kept in the fridge and consumed within three days of opening then that is what we should do.

CHAPTER 16

Processed Food and Additives

WHY DOES FOOD HAVE TO BE PROCESSED?

There are two main reasons for processing food. The first is to make certain kinds of food easier to eat. For example, cereal grains like wheat are very difficult to chew and digest, but once ground into flour, mixed with water and yeast, and baked into bread, they become readily palatable.

The second reason is to preserve it. In order to understand the importance of preserving food, think back to the Industrial Revolution when Britain had the misfortune of being the first country to become heavily industrialised. As more and more people deserted the land to begin a new life in the cities, it became necessary to find ways of feeding them. In those days when the distribution and transport systems were nowhere near as effective as they are today, it was difficult to get fresh food to the population in the cities before it went off. This created a very strong incentive to develop methods of preserving food – milk as cheese, fresh fruit as jam and so on. As most of the moulds and bacteria which cause food to go off cannot grow in high concentrations of sugar and salt, more and more came to be added to food so that it could be kept longer. Sugar is used as a preservative in jam but in most foods it is simply there to make them taste sweet.

Nowadays, with a steady stream of fresh fruit and vegetables being imported all year from around the world, kept fresh by refrigeration and rapidly distributed to every town in Britain, the need for processed food is far less than it used to be. Even with food grown in Britain, like potatoes and cabbages, the period during which it is available fresh is much longer than it used to be owing to the development of high yielding varieties which mature at different times of the year, and of improved storage facilities and methods. So we are rarely short of even home grown, fresh vegetables.

The same applies to dairy products. The development of high yielding breeds of cattle which can produce a thousand gallons of milk in the ten months after giving birth to a calf means that abundant supplies of fresh milk are now available. It can be kept refrigerated on the farm until collected and transported into the heart of the cities while it is still fresh, preferably after having most of the fat skimmed off of course. Hence there is no longer the same need for cheese or butter. There may still be a demand from people who like cheese and butter but not the same need.

Also technological developments which we now take for granted, like ultra-heat treatment to kill off micro-organisms, and the sealed cardboard carton which prevents micro-organisms from subsequently entering until it is opened, mean that milk is now available all the year round even in the most remote areas far from where it is produced. So too is fruit juice.

Food processing started out as an essential means of getting food to the people in the cities and ensuring that everyone had something to eat in the winter when fresh food was scarce, and I have nothing against processed food as such, so long as it still serves a useful purpose. After all, the wholemeal bread I keep encouraging everyone to eat more of is processed flour, and I can recommend eating lots of breakfast cereals, frozen mixed vegetables and cans of oily fish. The processed foods lining the shelves of your local supermarket vary from the wholesome, to products which are basically a mixture of colours and flavours with virtually no nutritional value at all.

Processed food can be good, bad or indifferent depending on the reason why it is processed, what is added during the processing, and the nutrient value of the food after it has been processed. The problem arises when colourings and flavourings, and sugar, salt and fat are added to processed foods in unnecessarily large amounts, without serving any useful purpose, other than perhaps to boost sales amongst those people who like the taste of the additives.

The only way of dealing with processed food is to Read That Label! Treat your supermarket as a bookshop and browse before you buy.

READY PREPARED MEALS

An extreme form of processing is the production of ready prepared meals. Such meals are a minefield. I came across a classic example in a major outlet recently: 'Salmon in a rich creamy sauce.' The healthiest of foods plastered with the most unhealthy. The Wimbledon strawberries and cream mentality revisited!

It is very easy to exceed your 30 gram per day limit of saturated fat by eating a single ready made meal and the pastry in a ready made pie. Take great care to read the labels before purchasing, keeping a wary eye on the fat and sugar content, as well as on the additives. Remember to take into account the fact that although the amount of fat in 100 grams may not seem too high, the size of the helping is usually about three times that. Marks and Spencer's Macaroni Cheese for example contains 10 grams of fat in every 100 grams, six of which are saturated. That may not sound too bad in itself, but eat a whole 283gm pack and that is 17gm of saturated fat. Add on the fat in the pastry of a fruit pie and you have exceeded the daily feed limit.

Any effort to provide some rough guidelines regarding the best ready prepared meals is complicated by the fact that the nutritional content of the same dish can vary so enormously between brands. Safeway's Macaroni Cheese, for example, contains less than half the total fat (4.5gm) and less than half the saturated fat (2.7gm) of the M & S meal without being advertised as a healthy option.

Not all Marks and Spencer's meals are full of fat. At the other extreme we have their haddock and chips and peas meal which has only one per cent fat.

SAUCES

To make the ready made meals more palatable you may wish to add some sauce to them. Again there is a bewildering array to choose from in the average supermarket. From the fat point of view, products vary enormously. At the one extreme is tomato ketchup which contains virtually no fat at all, and at the other, mayonnaise which is about three quarters fat, albeit mostly unsaturated. Some sauces have no additives, others are loaded with them. As always, it is worth spending a little time reading the labels to find out which is the best buy.

ADDITIVES: THE GOOD, THE BAD AND THE UGLY

Ideally additives should only be used if they confer some nutritional advantage on the food, like preserving it. One type of additive which serves no nutritionally useful purpose is colourings. On the contrary, the addition of colourings is often designed to encourage us to eat nutritionally poor quality food like sweets. The situation is more complicated with the colourings added to canned vegetables as it could be argued that they are there to encourage us to eat an otherwise healthy food.

CRACKING THE E CODE

When you cast your eye over the list of ingredients on a food label, the additives often look completely incomprehensible, just a jumble of numbers and meaningless names. What, for instance, do these strange looking numbers which begin with the letter E stand for? The aim of this chapter is to try and find our way through the additive maze, so that we can easily find out what is added to the food we are buying and what the various additives are there for.

Let us begin with the mysterious E numbers. The E numbers are a sort of universal language for use within the Common Market. Taking E110 to begin with; this is the code for a dye called sunset yellow which gives the yellow colour to yellow Smarties. French, German and other languages will all have their own words for sunset yellow, but the E number will be the same in France and Germany and the other countries as it is in Britain. The standard system of E numbers for permitted additives therefore makes it easier to move foods from country to country within the Common Market. British manufacturers are not obliged to use E numbers for goods destined for sale in Britain and some make life easier for us by just using the name of the substance.

Below I have produced a list of the most common additives used in Britain, so that when you see an E number you don't recognise, you can look it up in the list and find out what it is and what it does, and whether it might be harmful or not. We will start with the colourings as these have the lowest E numbers.

COLOURINGS

Many of the processed foods on the supermarket shelves contain colourings. They are used for a variety of reasons - to replace colour lost during processing or storage, to create an illusion of freshness, to make otherwise boring products look more attractive, especially to children, or to create 'new' products.

The natural colour of fruit and vegetables tends to be lost during the canning process owing to the high temperatures required to ensure that bacteria, especially the dreaded *Clostridium botulinum* – that name always sends a shiver down my spine – which is responsible for the potentially lethal form of food poisoning, botulism, are killed. Colours are therefore added to most canned food to replace that which has been lost; for example a green dye is added to peas to make them look green instead of brown, the manufacturers believing that we wouldn't buy their peas if they were the wrong colour. Are they correct?

Natural colours tend to fade with time anyway, and anything stored in clear glass bottles like fruit squash will lose its natural colour after it has been on the shelves for a while exposed to the light. So, to give food that fresh look, the manufacturers of squashes, like the manufacturers of curtains, use colour-fast, artificial dyes instead.

Manufacturers like colours and flavours because they enable them to create 'new' products. Adding different flavours to, for example, potato crisps makes it possible to extend their range, the idea being that if they have five different flavours they will sell more crisps in total than if they only had one flavour. Similarly if all of the sachets of blancmange in a box were of the same colour and flavour, customers might get bored, so they provide half a dozen different colours. There is nutritionally only one basic product but the addition of colours and flavours creates the illusion of variety and choice and therefore encourages us to eat and buy more.

Some colourings such as those with the numbers E160 to E163 occur naturally. They are what give the colour to, for instance, carrots, red peppers and beetroot and for use in the food industry are extracted from these and other plants. In the case of some other colourings which occur naturally, it is more economical to make them artificially in the laboratory. In such cases the 'artificial' substance is identical to the natural.

There are currently 20 permitted truly artificial colours. The two major groups of these artificial chemical dyes used in food colouring are the azo dyes and coal tar dyes which, as everyone knows, have been implicated in causing allergies and hyperactivity in children. Having said that, I have tried Smarties and they don't do a thing for me! So let us go through the list and see what we have.

If you want to play about with coal tar dyes, they can actually be bought in bottles as food colourings on the home baking section. Amongst those you can buy are erythrosine (pink-red); carmoisine (red); tartrazine (yellow), sunset yellow, and ponceau (red). They are great for giving your pumpkin a colourful glow at Halloween, but most people would certainly think twice before adding them to food that is to be eaten.

Baby foods are only allowed to contain the natural colours like carotene and riboflavin which are also vitamins, so the only way to be sure of avoiding artificial colourings is to eat nothing but baby food! I am joking, of course!

To get us into a good mood, let us start off with two natural orange-yellow colourings.

E100 Curcumin
This is a natural orange-yellow colouring which is extracted from a tropical plant known as turmeric. It is used to restore the yellow colour to butter, processed cheese and margarine as well as being found in ice cream, fish fingers, curry powder, savoury rice and so on.

E101 Riboflavin
That name sounds familiar. Yes, of course, it is none other than our old friend vitamin B2. Hi, there! As well as being used as a vitamin supplement in breakfast cereals, it is added to sauces and processed cheese to impart an orange-yellow colour.

Now we are on to the artificial azo dyes. In those people who are allergic to the azo dyes they can produce skin irritation, symptoms reminiscent of hay fever and breathing difficulties, blurred vision, purple patches on the skin. Those who are sensitive to aspirin, or who suffer from asthma or eczema seem to be most at risk. Azo dyes are also suspected of causing hyperactivity in children. They are easy to spot from their E numbers as they all lie between E102 and E155.

THE YELLOW PERIL
E102 Tartrazine
Tartrazine, the best known of the azo dyes, is added to a wide range of products to impart a yellow colour including biscuits, cakes, chewing gum, custard powder, fish fingers, fizzy drinks, fruit squash, jellies, and tinned vegetables.

E104 Quinoline Yellow
This is a greenish-yellow coal tar dye which is added to such products as cake mixes, ice cream, lemon-flavoured

foods, fruit squash, fizzy drinks, Scotch eggs and smoked haddock. It has been associated with hyperactivity in children.

E110 Sunset Yellow
An azo dye which is added to cakes, cake mix, custard powder, fish fingers, ice cream, lemon-flavoured foods, fruit squash, jam.

SEEING RED
The first on our red list is a natural colouring, but the rest are azo dyes.

E120 Cochineal
Prepared from insects, it is expensive to produce so is not widely used, but it can be found in some alcoholic drinks, biscuits, cakes and icing. As it comes from insects,vegetarians may wish to avoid it.

E123 Amaranth
This purple-red azo dye is one of the most widely used colourings and is found in such products as cakes, fruit squash, ice cream, medicines, and soup.

E124 Ponceau 4R
An azo dye, widely used to colour foods red. It is banned in America and Norway. It is added to cake, cake mix, custard powder, jam, jellies, milk shakes, sauces and soup.

E127 Erythrosine
A coal tar dye used to colour foods pink or red. It used to be more widely used, but because it contains iodine which in large amounts could affect the thyroid gland of children, its use in Britain is now confined mainly to glacé and cocktail cherries and Scotch eggs.

E128 Red 2G
An artificial red azo dye used to impart a red colour to some jams, milk shakes and sausages. It is banned in most European countries, Australia, Japan and North America.

GETTING THE BLUES
Two blues, both coal tar dyes which can produce allergic reaction in susceptible individuals and have been associated with hyperactivity in children.

E131 Patent Blue
Used for imparting a blue colour to ice cream, Scotch eggs, sweets.

E132 Indigo Carmine
Amongst the products it is added to are biscuits, cake decorations, Swiss roll, sweets.

TURNING GREEN
E133 Brilliant Blue FCF
A synthetic blue coal tar dye frequently used with the yellow dye tartrazine to produce various shades of green. It is added to some fizzy drinks and is used to return the green colour to mint sauce and canned processed peas. It is banned in most European countries.

E140 and E141 Chlorophyll and Chlorophyllins
A natural olive green colour extracted from plants. Hopefully the solvents used for extracting it have all been removed. It is added to, for instance, ice cream and soups.

THE RICH DARK BROWN LOOK OF CHOCOLATE AND GRAVY
The food painter is able to recreate this using the dyes

below:

E150 Caramel
Large amounts of caramel are used in soft drinks especially Cola, and it is added to some beers, meat products and soups. In order to give the impression that their chocolate biscuits are brimming over with chocolate some manufacturers use caramel blended with amaranth to give a rich chocolate appearance. To give the impression that they are full of meat, sausage casings may be dipped in caramel to obtain the desired colour. Some brown bread is simply white bread to which caramel has been added to make it look brown.

E151 Black PN
An artificial purple-black coal tar dye which is added to brown sauce, chocolate mousse, gravy.

E153 Carbon Black
Carbon black is produced from burnt plant material. It is banned in America owing to fears that handling the dye during manufacture could cause skin cancer. It is added to chocolate-flavoured foods, jam and liquorice.

E154 Brown FK
This artificial, yellow-brown, coal tar dye is added to kippers and other smoked fish, gravy, and to give a browned look to cooked chicken. It is banned in America and some European countries.

E155 Brown HT
This artificial brown coal tar dye is added to chocolate-flavoured foods. It is banned in America and some European countries.

BACK TO NATURE

As we have seen, not all colourings are artificial dyes. Some are extracted naturally from plants. These are now being widely used in children's drinks and other foods as an alternative to the coal tar dyes. For example, Stripes milk drink made with semi-skimmed milk comes in several flavours. To give the banana flavour a yellowish colour the manufacturers add the natural colourings turmeric and annatto; to give the strawberry flavour a reddish colour, they add the natural dye carmine (derived from cochineal); while to give the chocolate flavour a chocolate colour they use the real thing, cocoa powder. When the drinks come in small cardboard cartons to be drunk through a plastic straw it is difficult to see the point of adding any colourings at all as you can't see what the colour is anyway. However, the natural colourings are a definite improvement on the synthetic colourings which might have been used in the past.

The colourings listed below are extracted from plants. Some processed foods which used to contain coal tar dyes can now be bought coloured with these instead.

E160(a) Carotenes

This is the family of our old friend beta-carotene which, as you know, our bodies can convert into vitamin A. They give the yellow colour to carrots, peppers, tomatoes and other deeply coloured vegetables. The products they are added to include custard, margarine, processed cheese, rice pudding, salad dressing.

E160(b) Annatto, Bixin, Norbixin

These are the various aliases of a yellow colouring made from the seed pods of the annatto tree. It is often used as a safer alternative to tartrazine. OK so long as the chemicals used in its extraction are removed. It is added to cheese, custard, ice cream, fish fingers, salad cream.

PRESERVATIVES

As preservatives slow down the growth of moulds, fungi and bacteria which would otherwise cause the food to go off, their addition is more morally defensible than that of colourings. Even more importantly, they help to prevent harmful bacteria which cause food poisoning from growing on it. The most serious form of food poisoning is botulism which is caused by an organism called *Clostridium botulinum.* If allowed to grow on food it produces a very dangerous toxin, which remains poisonous even if the food is subsequently heated to a high enough temperature to kill the bacteria. Preservatives are essential, therefore, if we are to continue to enjoy certain kinds of food. On the minus side, some can provoke allergies, and there are concerns about the long-term safety of some of them.

Preservatives are easy to spot on the list of E numbers because they all have numbers between E200 and E297.

PREVENTING FOOD FROM GOING MOULDY

E200-E203 Sorbic acid and sorbates

Sorbic acid occurs naturally in some fruit and berries, but that used by the food industry is usually produced synthetically. It slows down the growth of moulds and yeasts and is added to a wide variety of foods including cake, cheese spread, frozen pizza, fruit pie, soft drinks, cider and wine.

E210- E213 Benzoic acid and benzoates

Benzoic acid is used to prevent the growth of bacteria and is also effective against some moulds. It is added to a wide variety of foods, particularly those which contain fruit like soft drinks, jam, pickles, sauces, as well as in yoghurt and margarine.

E214-E219 Hydroxybenzoates
These are used to prevent the growth of yeasts and moulds. They are added to jam, pie filling, pickles, salad cream and soft drinks.

E220 Sulphur dioxide
Sulphur dioxide is one of the most widely used additives as it has several different functions. As well as being used as a fungicide to prevent fruit from going mouldy, it is used to prevent cut fruit from going brown; as an antioxidant for fat and oil products; and as a bleaching agent for flour. It is therefore very difficult to avoid. It turns up in alcoholic drinks, desserts, jams and marmalade, jellies, fruit juices, pickles, dried fruit, soups, spices and vegetables, to name just a few.

E221-E227 Sulphites and Metabisulphites
As well as being used as a preservative, they are used to sterilise equipment, as an antioxidant and to slow down the browning process in apples and potatoes. They are added to alcoholic drinks, frozen chips, frozen seafood, fruit juice, orange squash, pickles.

E230-E233 Biphenyls
These E numbers are not likely to be found on labels, as biphenyls are used to prevent the growth of moulds on the outside of citrus fruit. It is either applied directly to the skin or to the paper that is used for wrapping them. If the skin of citrus fruit is to be used in a recipe, it should be washed in detergent first and then rinsed thoroughly.

E234 Nisin

Nisin is an antibiotic produced by a particular strain of the *Streptococcus* bacterium which, like many bacteria and moulds, produces antibiotics to kill or slow down the growth of other kinds of bacteria and moulds. Some, like penicillin from the bread mould *Penicillium*, have been exploited by medical science. There are bloody battles raging on a typical slice of mouldy bread! Nisin is produced naturally by the micro-organisms in some cheeses and may be added as a preservative to other cheeses and cheese spreads and some canned foods.

THE DREADED BOTULISM

E249 and E250 Potassium nitrite and Sodium nitrite

These are artificially produced preservatives, which are used as curing agents for meat. Their most important function is to prevent the growth of the bacterium which causes botulism, the most serious form of food poisoning. They are used in meat products, such as pork pies and sausages. There is some evidence that they could react in the stomach with other chemicals called amines to produce new chemicals which might increase the risk of cancer. They are banned from food produced specifically for babies.

E251 and E252 Sodium nitrate and Potassium nitrate

They have much the same uses as the nitrites above, and can be converted into them, so the health risks are also similar.

SOME MORE COMMON ANTI-MOULD WEAPONRY

E260 Acetic acid

This is simply the scientific name for vinegar which is used in pickles to prevent the growth of bacteria and moulds.

E261 Potassium acetate
A preservative used in frozen vegetables and bread.

E262 Sodium dihydrogen acetate
This is mainly used to prevent bacteria from growing in bread and as a flavouring in crisps.

E263 Calcium acetate
Used to prevent mould growing in bread. Also found in jelly and cake mix.

E270 Lactic acid
Lactic acid is produced in milk when it turns sour. Amongst the food it is added to are beer, bread, cheese, fizzy drinks and margarine.

E280-E283 Propionic acid and Propionates
Propionic acid is added to bread to prevent the growth of moulds.

E290 Carbon dioxide
Best known for putting the fizz into fizzy drinks, this gas, which is naturally present in the air we breathe, is also used as a preservative.

E296 Malic acid
Used to regulate acidity in foods and as a flavouring. It is added to packet and tinned soup, mince meats, jam, frozen vegetables, and savoury rice.

E297 Fumaric acid
Also used to regulate acidity, and is added to cake mix, jam, soft drinks, jellies and sweets.

PREVENTING FATS AND OILS FROM TURNING RANCID

In contact with the oxygen of the air, fats and oils soon become rancid. Antioxidants are substances which help to prevent this from happening and also prevent the deterioration of fat soluble vitamins in food.

E300-E304 Ascorbic acid

You may have noticed 'ascorbic acid' written on bread labels or powdered milk cartons and meat products. Ascorbic acid is the scientific name for our old friend, vitamin C. This is therefore an extremely natural additive recruited here for its antioxidant properties rather than as an intentional vitamin supplementation.

E306-E309 Tocopherols

Better known as vitamin E the tocopherols are commonly used as an antioxidant in meat pies and vegetable fats and oils.

E310 to E312 Gallates

These are purely synthetic chemicals. They are banned from food prepared specifically for babies but used in vegetable oils, margarine, instant mashed potato and some breakfast cereals.

E320 and E321 Butylated Hydroxyanisole and Butylated Hydroxytoluene

These antioxidants are commonly added to margarine, cooking fats and vegetable oil and to fatty foods like chips and crisps. They are used in a wide range of foods from cheese spreads to biscuits. Citric acid is often used with them to promote their action. They can cause an allergic reaction in people sensitive to them, and are banned from foods prepared specifically for babies.

EMULSIFIERS, STABILISERS, THICKENING AGENTS AND SEQUESTRANTS

E322-E927

As these are usually listed on labels by name rather than by E number, I will avoid confusing the issue by giving E numbers you are hardly ever likely to come across. A brief word first about what these substances do. Emulsifiers are used to bind together oil and water into an emulsion. A familiar example is the use of an egg to make a mayonnaise or to bind a sauce, when the lethicin in the egg is acting as an emulsifier. Like lethicin, many emulsifiers are natural substances.

The purpose of stabilisers is to keep oil and water together and to counteract their natural tendency to separate.

Thickening agents are used to bulk out food and to make it look more solid. Many substances used as stabilisers and thickeners occur naturally. They include agar and carrageenan produced from seaweed; locust bean gum extracted from pods of the locust or carob tree; guar gum extracted from pea seeds; tragacanth and gum arabic extracted from trees found in the Middle East; xanthum gum, a by-product of corn syrup fermentation; karaya gum extracted from trees found in South East Asia; and pectin extracted from the leftovers of oranges and apples used in the production of orange juice and cider.

FLAVOURINGS

Most processed foods as well as having colours added to them also have added flavourings. It is of course the taste and flavour of food which gives it its special appeal; without its natural flavourings our food wouldn't be the same. Just imagine the glorious aroma of freshly baked bread emanating from the bakery behind the bread counter and the smells emanating from an oriental restaurant, guaranteed to get the digestive juices moving, or the familiar smell of burnt toast which stimulates not only the taste buds but also the ear with its accompaniment of a wailing smoke detector.

Most flavours are volatile and unstable and easily lost when food is stored. Reheated food rarely tastes as good as it did when first prepared. In large-scale manufacture, such as that needed to get soup into cans and onto a supermarket shelf, much of the original flavour of the food is lost. The only answer is for the manufacturer to add the flavour – or something resembling it – back again.

There are about 2,000 different flavours commonly added to food in the UK. The good news is that about nine out of ten of these are naturally occurring substances extracted from plants. Most of the remainder are identical to natural flavours, but are made artificially in the laboratory simply because it is cheaper and easier than extracting them from their natural source.

Unlike food colourings which tend to be a single substance like beta-carotene, or sunset yellow, most things described as a flavour on a packet or bottle of processed food are a mixture of different chemicals. Cherry flavour for instance is likely to consist of about a dozen different flavours mixed together in the correct proportions, to produce something which tastes vaguely like cherries. It's a skilful job mixing all these flavours together to get the taste and smell you want, like creating a new perfume or blend of whisky.

Flavours do not have E numbers and there is not the same amount of control exerted over them as there is with colours. New flavours are not subjected to the same rigorous testing as a new colouring or a new drug would be. This is not quite so alarming as it might sound because our taste buds are extremely sensitive organs and the amount of a flavour which needs to be added to food is incredibly small, so small in most cases that it is difficult to see how they could be harmful. The average person only consumes about a teaspoonful of artificially manufactured flavours a year. This is not to say that we should be complacent as there may be flavours lurking out there somewhere which are harmful in minute amounts. Regulations are at last being drawn up to begin to control the addition of flavours to foods.

If we take on board the main message of this book and concentrate on eating the best of fresh foods that the supermarket has to offer, and less processed, we will reduce our consumption of colours and flavours without really trying.

HIGH SALT: HIGH BLOOD PRESSURE

The additive of most concern to many people is salt, excessive consumption of salt being a major factor contributing to raised blood pressure. Most people in Britain consume more salt than is good for them with the result that the average blood pressure of the British population is higher than it need be. Although two out of three people still add salt to their cooking this contributes only a small part to the total salt in our diet.

Ordinary table salt is sodium chloride. Most foods also contain another kind of salt, potassium chloride, which does not have the same affect on blood pressure as the sodium salt.

Virtually all natural food, including unprocessed cereal grains, fruit and vegetables and wild game contain more potassium than sodium, so for millions of years people have been eating more potassium than sodium. Today in Britain, however, most of us consume more sodium than potassium and that is the main reason the

British tend to have higher blood pressures than people of similar age in those parts of the world where salt consumption is lower.

Why is it then, if almost every kind of fresh food contains more potassium than sodium, that most of us in this country get it the wrong way round and eat more sodium than potassium?

The reason will come as no surprise. It is the obvious one that so much of the food we eat isn't fresh at all. It's processed. Cornflakes, for example, have over 1,000 times as much sodium as the fresh corn they are made from.

It is the same with most breakfast cereals although, despite the salt, cereals are still a good, energy rich, low fat food, full of B vitamins so, unless you are under doctor's orders to cut down on salt, just keep enjoying them. Some have less salt than others though. Weetabix, for instance, has only a third as much sodium in every 100 grams as Cornflakes.

It is much the same story for most other foods. Crisps typically have 100 times more sodium than the same amount of baked potato. And canned vegetables and soups nearly all have loads of salt added to them. So do cans of luncheon meat, as well as the processed meats on the meat counter, and don't forget salted butter and cheese. Avoiding high salt products like these is especially important for people who have high blood pressure, and the elderly.

We need to keep up the pressure on the food manufacturers to keep our blood pressure down by using no more sodium salt in their products than is absolutely necessary.

To make matters even worse, during the processing most of the potassium gets leached out.

Read That Label before buying processed foods to find out how much salt they contain. Cans of baked beans are a classic example. As we saw in our visit to the vegetable section, in any supermarket you will find different brands of baked beans standing side by side on the shelf, some with half the amount of salt (and less sugar) than those next to them.

BEFORE YOU BUY, READ THAT LABEL AND CHOOSE THE HEALTHY OPTION

That is the way to shop. Look before you buy! Read That Label! Why buy a less healthy product when an identical healthier option is sitting on the shelf right next to it? You find this all the time – virtually identical products side by side on the shelf, but one of which has more salt or more fat or more sugar added to it. Always go for the healthy option. It takes a little more time initially to read the labels and compare brands, but once you have worked out which is the healthier option you can head straight for it next time.

NOT ALL BAD

Despite their bad press, it becomes clear that not all additives are bad for us. As we have seen, they are not all the artificial, way out things like the coal tar dyes in sweeties. Some additives are even positively beneficial in themselves like E300, vitamin C.

Ideally, all of the food we eat should be fresh and there should be no need for preservatives but this is a situation which in practice is very difficult to achieve. In general, the health risk associated with food infested with moulds and bacteria is likely to be greater than that associated with the careful use of preservatives. On the other hand the safety of certain preservatives, like nitrites, does cause some concern, and we are always wise to choose the fresh option when there is one available.

Sugar and salt are the most common additives which

are widely used in the preservation of food. Jam for instance would soon go mouldy if it wasn't for the high concentration of sugar it contains. But excessive amounts of salt and sugar, as you know, are not healthy. Too much salt can result in high blood pressure and too much sugar in tooth decay and obesity. So their use is valuable, in fact essential, if we are to continue eating certain types of food, but we should avoid consuming excessive amounts of them.

When there is a good reason for additives and they have been proven to be safe I have no argument with them. What I don't like is additives being used simply for cosmetic reasons, to create pretty colours in sweets, for example, or to give horrid flavours to fizzy drinks. Almost all of the added colours and flavours have absolutely no nutritional value. Although some are completely natural substances, others are completely unnatural and may even be harmful to people who are susceptible to them. It makes sense, therefore, to avoid as far as possible products which have too many unnecessary colours added to them. As a general rule, the more heavily processed a food is, the more additives it is likely to contain.

CHAPTER 17

Food Safety: How to Avoid Food Poisoning

Outbreaks of food poisoning as a result of supermarket produce are surprisingly rare when you consider the incredible number of products on sale and their diverse origins. It is all down to the very careful adherence to rules governing the preparation and storage of products by manufacturers, suppliers, and supermarkets alike. It would be a pity after all of this trouble has been taken by the supermarkets on our behalf, if once the food was in our possession, we dropped our guard and allowed it to become contaminated with bacteria. More so, if we then let them grow unchecked and poison us.

The first step is to ensure that we always use unpackaged food as soon as possible and packaged food by the 'use by' date on the label, or sooner if we are unable to adhere to the manufacturer's storage instructions. If, for example, the label states that the product should be stored at 0-5°C, but we don't have a refrigerator, then it should be kept in a cool place and preferably consumed on the day of purchase.

WHAT CAUSES FOOD POISONING?

The most common type of food poisoning is caused by bacteria being inadvertently allowed to grow on food, usually meat products. Some kinds of bacteria, of which

**Big Jock Horner,
Sat in a dirty corner,
Eating his cold meat pie,
He caught Salmonella,
Unfortunate Fella,
And now he feels like
he is going to die.**

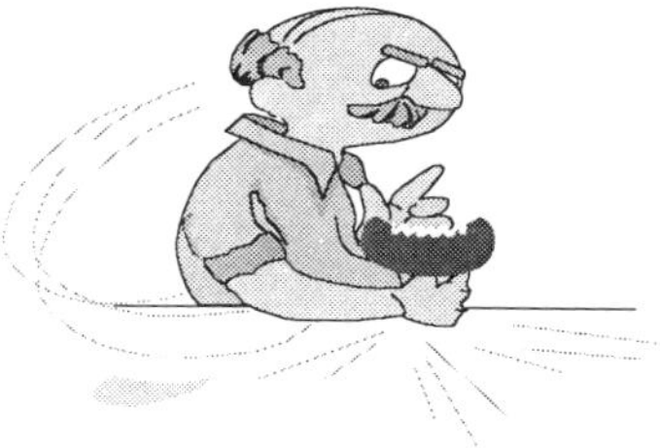

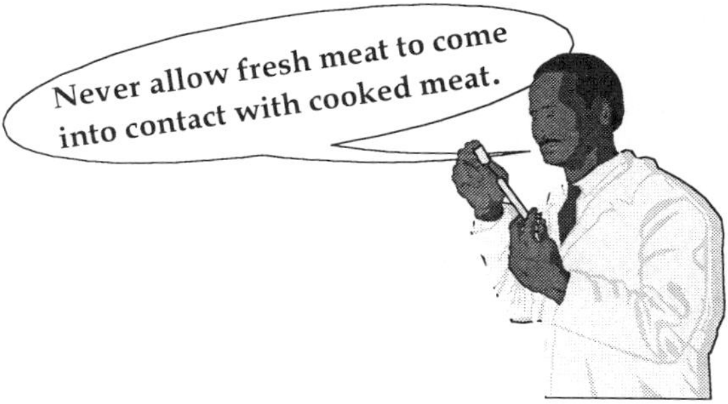

the best known is *Salmonella,* can if consumed along with our food, take up temporary residence in our intestines, increase vastly in numbers and produce an unpleasant infection. Others types of bacteria, like *Staphylococcus,* have a different strategy. As they grow on meat, they produce toxins, and it is these toxins, rather than the bacteria themselves, which make us ill.

The bacteria may be in the meat already or they may be transferred to it from other meat or from the skin of those working with the meat.

HOW TO AVOID FOOD POISONING

1. Prevent food from becoming contaminated in the first place

Once we have purchased our meat and poultry, we should wrap it separately to prevent one piece of meat coming into contact with another, especially fresh meat and poultry from coming into contact with ready-to-eat meat.

When we arrive home with our purchases, we should ensure that the fresh meat or poultry does not contaminate anything ready to eat that is already in the fridge. In case there are any drips, raw meat, or food that is defrosting, should be kept near the bottom underneath any cooked food, and both should be covered. If we buy free-range eggs from the local farm we should take just as much care not to let them come into contact with other products and to cook them thoroughly before eating.

If we chop up fresh meat, remember that the chopping board and knife and our fingers may be contaminated with bacteria from the meat so we should wash all of them before using them again for handling other foods.

Needless to say, hands should always be washed after going to the lavatory and handling pets, and pets which may previously have had their noses in something unpleasant should be kept away. Faeces, both human and animal, are a potent source of *Salmonella* which may be transferred to food via unwashed hands, dogs' noses or flies' feet. Eggs of course may be contaminated directly by the birds which laid them. Tortoises and turtles are usually infected with nasty strains of *Salmonella* so if you have any of these pets around be sure to wash your hands thoroughly after handling them. The biggest menace of all are human carriers of *Salmonella* and other harmful gut bacteria who fail to wash their hands after going to the lavatory and thereby manage to initiate large-scale outbreaks of food poisoning amongst the customers of the canteens, restaurants and shops where they work.

2. Cool it!

The second line of defence is to keep meat products at a low temperature and consume them as soon as possible before bacteria have a chance to grow. If the meat is deep frozen, bacteria, even if present in it, cannot increase in numbers. At a normal fridge temperature of 0-5°C they multiply very slowly, if at all. At room temperature they multiply much faster and next to a central heating radiator, or in the boot of a car on a warm day, they can really get going.

When doing the week's shopping in the supermarket, chilled and frozen foods should be bought last so that they have less time to thaw out before we get them home and safely into the fridge. If we will not be heading home immediately, it is a good idea, if they are to be left in the warm boot of a car for any length of time, to use a cool bag or box with ice cubes.

The good news: cooking kills bacteria

The good news is that thoroughly cooking food will kill *Salmonella* and most other bacteria so long as the oven is preheated thoroughly and the cooking times on food labels adhered to. Take special care with large pieces of frozen meat and poultry. If it isn't thawed all of the way through, the centre may not be cooked enough. As in poultry, the centre is where most of the bacteria are, and that is not good news. The best way to thaw food is either in the refrigerator or in a microwave, as leaving it for too long in a warm room may allow its temperature to rise to a point where the bacteria can start increasing in numbers.

Food cooked for eating later should be cooled as quickly as possible in a cold place, and once it is cool, placed in the fridge. Placing it in the fridge straight-away might increase the temperature of the fridge and encourage the growth of bacteria on the food that is already there. Raw eggs sometimes contain food poisoning bacteria and are best cooked.

The bad news: cooking doesn't necessarily kill the toxins produced by bacteria

The bad news is that toxins produced by bacteria such as *Staphylococcus* and *Clostridia* may not be destroyed by cooking.

The most serious kind of food poisoning is botulism caused by the bacterium *Clostridium botulinum*. Clostridium is what is known as an anaerobic bacterium. What this means is that it can grow in the absence of air, for example in a sealed can. Boiling up the contents of the can after we open it may kill the bacterium but not the deadly toxin it produces. It is because of *Clostridium botulinum* that manufacturers have to heat food put into cans to such a high temperature that they lose their colour and much of their texture. Unlike most bacteria, such as *Salmonella,* which are easily killed by moderate temperatures such as those used in pasteurising milk,

Clostridium produces spores which can only be destroyed by exposure to very high temperatures. The heat resistant spores combined with the heat resistant toxins make *Clostridium* the food technologist's worst enemy

There is comparatively little we can do to protect ourselves against botulism. Our life is in the hands of the manufacturers.

Protecting at-risk groups of people

When preparing food for young children, pregnant women, the very elderly or anyone with low resistance to infection, we should be extra careful. Eggs should be cooked thoroughly until both the yolk and whites are solid and any ready cooked, chilled meals or ready-to-eat poultry that we buy should *not* be regarded as ready to eat until they have been re-cooked. For most of us, most of the time, such extreme precautions are not necessary.

To avoid the risk of *Listeria,* women while they are pregnant should avoid eating soft ripened cheeses of the brie, camembert or blue-vein types.

Not all bacteria which contaminate food do us any harm. For instance, we can usually tolerate a small dose of a type of bacteria called *E coli,* as it lives happily in all of our guts anyway. Unfortunately, from time to time virulent strains of such normally harmless bacteria can turn up. *E coli 157* is a notable example, which has caused serious long-term illness in some children who have become infected. Contamination with such organisms can only be avoided if all along the line, from manufacturer to consumer, all of the basic safety precautions are strictly adhered to.

Don't overdo the cooking!

Although meat products and poultry should be cooked thoroughly to kill bacteria so that we avoid food poisoning, it is equally important not to overdo the roasting or grilling. It is a wise precaution to avoid eating anything that is obviously burnt, whether it is meat or toast, as burning food generates a cocktail of obnoxious chemicals some of which may be as potentially harmful as those in cigarette smoke. If you come across any burnt bits, cut them off and display them in a prominent position so that the cook gets the hint!

The Healthy Eating Pyramid

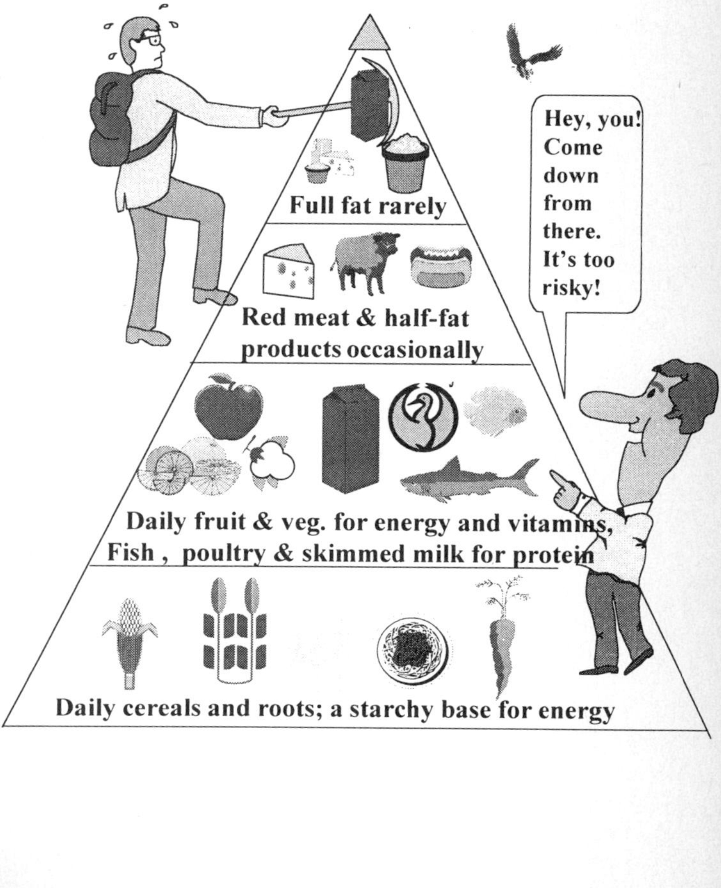

CHAPTER 18

The Healthy Eating Pyramid and a Healthy Varied Diet

OK, now if you are feeling fit it's time to draw up a Healthy Eating Pyramid. First draw a big triangle to represent a pyramid and draw three lines through it to separate it into four levels. At the base of the pyramid we will start off with those foods we need to eat every day to provide us with the bulk of our energy to keep us going. On the level above that we will place other foods which we also need to eat lots of, to provide us with the protein and extra vitamins we need to stay healthy. In the middle, we will list the food that can be eaten occasionally as a special treat, but not every day. Finally at the top of the pyramid we will place those foods which are bad for us and which we should therefore eat as little of as possible.

THE STARCHY BASE OF THE PYRAMID

The pyramid needs a firm base so, let us start with the kind of food we should eat lots of every day. Which foods are an especially good source of energy first of all?

The answer is starchy foods, and that means bread, especially wholemeal bread, potatoes and other root vegetables, breakfast cereals, rice and pasta.

They also contain lots of protein, B vitamins, minerals and fibre.

THE EQUALLY HEALTHY SECOND LEVEL

For the second level, we are looking for foods we can eat practically every day to provide us with extra protein and vitamins in addition to that in the starchy foods.

For first-class protein, we should eat poultry, fish and wild game like venison, semi-skimmed or skimmed milk, cottage cheese, low fat yoghurt and egg whites. We should also eat peas and beans which, when combined with cereals, add up to top-quality protein.

For extra vitamins and minerals, fresh fruit like apples, pears and bananas, pure fruit juices, and fresh and frozen green vegetables are ideal.

THE THIRD LEVEL OF THE PYRAMID

The third level consists of those foods which can be eaten occasionally as a special treat but, because they contain too much fat or sugar, not in large amounts every day.

These include cakes, biscuits, sticky puddings, chocolates, crisps, chips, jam and marmalade, sweets, ice cream and half fat cheese. Always choose the low fat options when available.

The leaner cuts of red meat with the visible fat removed, and food fried in fresh vegetable oils, and nuts are also acceptable from time to time.

THE SLIPPERY TOP OF THE PYRAMID

Now for the top of the pyramid and foods we should eat as little of as possible, mainly because they contain too much saturated fat.

As we have emphasised throughout this guide, most pig, cow and sheep products contain far too much fat. The occasional 'lean' joint of red meat won't do us any harm but so as not to eat these products too often, we should steer clear of processed meats like sausages, meat pies, mince, burgers, and luncheon meats most of the time, just having one or two of them say once a week.

We should also avoid full fat dairy products like butter, cream, full fat milk and full fat cheese, and take semi-skimmed and skimmed milk and low fat cheeses instead.

There is no longer any excuse for frying food in lard and butter, a practice which should be completely abandoned in favour of vegetable oil, non-stick pans or alternative methods of cooking.

HEALTHY EATING MEANS INCREASED VARIETY, NOT LESS

Looking carefully at the pyramid, it becomes clear just how few forbidden foods there are. It is a common misconception that healthy eating means depriving ourselves. On the contrary, it simply means eating more of the healthy, interesting foods in the bottom layers of the pyramid and not so much of the high fat, high sugar and high salt products further up. More excitingly, it means keeping our eyes and ears open for new healthy items and recipes to enrich our eating.

Now that you are fully steeped in the principles of a healthy diet, as you come across other foods, you will know where they fit on the pyramid and whether they should be eaten regularly or sparingly.

HEALTHY FOOD IS NO DEARER THAN UNHEALTHY FOOD

Some people say that they don't eat healthy food because it's too expensive. In my view that argument against healthy eating is utter nonsense.

We all know that bread is cheaper than cake and biscuits. Poultry is cheaper than red meat. Today, fresh chicken was selling in the local Safeway for 95p per pound compared with silverside at £2.78p per pound.

Raw potatoes only cost about a tenth as much as the same weight of crisps and are much cheaper than chips. For a quick snack, an apple can be had for about half the price of a packet of crisps. Bread without butter or margarine is obviously cheaper than bread with butter or margarine. Tap water is cheaper than fizzy drinks full of flavours and additives and just about as nutritious. Potatoes, swedes, carrots, brown rice and pasta are all inexpensive sources of vitamins and energy-yielding carbohydrate. I could go on and on.

On the contrary, as you would expect, high fat, high salt, processed foods are usually more expensive than the same amount of fresh food owing to all of the time and effort – the production cost – which goes into the processing.

But what about healthy varieties of the same food; skimmed milk compared with full fat, or baked beans without added sugar compared with baked beans with added sugar? Let us make a simple comparison of supermarket prices of healthy compared with unhealthy varieties of particular foods and see if there is any difference. This is based on a recent visit to three local supermarkets. The particular supermarkets are chosen because they happen to have branches near where I live or work.

The table below confirms that the healthy option is usually no more expensive than the unhealthy. Two notable exceptions being half fat cheese and bread, the cheapest wholemeal usually selling for about a third more than the cheapest white loaves, although Asda had an exceptionally good priced wholemeal. On the other hand, standard breakfast cereals like Cornflakes usually cost about a third less than their sugary equivalents.

SUPERMARKET PRICES OF ORDINARY AND HEALTHY OPTIONS COMPARED

Product and size	Option	Asda	Safeway	Tesco
Fresh chicken (per kilogram)		£1.45	£2.09	£1.52
Silverside (per kilogram)		£6.65	£6.12	£7.23
Kellogg's Frosties (500g)	40% sugar	£1.59	£1.64	£1.64
Kellogg's Corn Flakes (500g)	8% sugar	£1.07	£1.09	£1.09
Milk (Safeway and	Full fat	25	28	28
Tesco 1pint, Asda 500ml)	Semi-skimmed	25	28	28
	Skimmed	25	28	28
Cheddar cheese: pre-packed	Full fat	£2.84	£3.49	£3.06
cheapest (per kilogram)	Half fat	£4.71	£5.46	£5.05
Soft cheese Philadelphia	Full fat	£1.19	84	89
(Safeway & Tesco 150g,	Light	£1.19	84	89
Asda 200g)				
Rice pudding Ambrosia	Full fat	45	45	45
(425g)	Low fat	45	45	45
Baked beans: Heinz (420g)	Ordinary	31	31	33
	Weight Watchers	31	31	31
Tinned peach slices:	In syrup	49	49	49
Del Monte (410g)	In juice	52	52	52
Tinned carrots	In salt	22	37	37
(Tesco, Safeways 400g; Asda 300g)	Without added salt	27	37	37
Digestive biscuits				
(400g) McVitie's	Ordinary	71 (500g)	63	59
(400g) McVitie's	25% less fat	63	63	63
(400g) Burton's	50% less fat	59	60	60
Cheapest bread	White	37	27	27

Wholemeal	39	48	49

Note: Supermarket prices vary weekly. This table should not be taken as indicating that one supermarket chain consistently offers better value than another.

THE VIRTUES OF A VARIED DIET

The most important thing to remember is that there is nothing better than a well-balanced diet. I am sure you will be convinced by now that healthy eating, far from being boring, opens up new opportunities, encouraging us to enrich our eating with new foods we hadn't tried before. The French, remember, have one of the healthiest diets in the world with one of the lowest rates of heart disease and French cuisine could hardly be described as boring.

Avoid at all cost those kamikaze diets which many people adhere to, like the Macho Man's Meat Pie, Chips and Lager Diet, or the Fat Ladies' Cake With Everything Diet, or the Kid's Crisps, Fizzy Drinks and Snack Bar Diet.

At the other extreme, we don't want to go overboard on anything and eat huge amounts of it to the exclusion of other foods just because we think it is particularly healthy. That is exactly what people did in the past with milk and butter and we definitely don't want to make that mistake again.

Eat plenty of fresh fruit, green vegetables, fish and poultry, drink semi-skimmed milk, and get most of your energy from starchy foods like root vegetables and cereals instead of from fatty foods like red meat, cake and biscuits and you won't go far wrong.

AND PLENTY OF REGULAR EXERCISE

We will benefit from healthy eating whether we take any exercise or not, but just think how much greater the benefit will be if our new healthier lifestyle includes lots of regular exercise as well. Like healthy eating, regular exercise has been shown to reduce the risk of coronary heart disease, high blood pressure and osteoporosis, and by burning off the excess calories helps us to avoid overweight and obesity. Lack of exercise is not just a British problem; it is estimated that half of the world's population now take too little exercise. Labour-saving devices in the home and in the workplace have greatly reduced the amount of regular daily exercise, and now that most people drive to work instead of walking, even to the bus stop, millions get virtually no exercise from one week to the next.

The World Health Organisation and the International Federation of Sports Medicine have got together to issue recommendations regarding the minimum amount of exercise we should be taking. These are published in the Bulletin of the World Health Organisation, 1995, page 136.

- Daily physical activity should be accepted as the cornerstone of a healthy lifestyle. Physical activity should be reintegrated into the routine of everyday living. An obvious first step would be the use of stairs instead of lifts, and walking or cycling for short journeys.
- Adults should be encouraged to increase habitual physical activity gradually, aiming to carry out every day at least 30 minutes of physical activity of moderate intensity. Eg brisk walking and stair climbing. More strenuous activities such as slow jogging, cycling, field and court games (soccer, tennis etc.) and swimming could provide additional benefits.
- The fact that there are benefits to be gained by starting physical activity at any age should be broadcast more widely.

Note carefully the words 'at least 30 minutes of physical activity'. There is no reason why we should not set our sights higher than this and aim for 30 minutes of vigorous activity at least twice a day. Many readers, particularly those of you who walk to work, will probably be taking this amount of exercise anyway and may wish to set your sights higher still to become even fitter.

At the opposite end of the spectrum, those who drive everywhere and are very unfit should start with gentle walking and build up gradually over a period of months using a programme such as that described in *Fitness Walking* by Les Snowdon and Maggie Humphreys, published by Mainstream in 1992.

Plenty of brisk walking, jogging, ball games, swimming, dancing, exercise classes, workouts to videos, weight training – whatever we enjoy doing – will help us to get the most out of all this good food.

CHAPTER 19

The Seek and Reduce Calorie and Fat Counter

A HAPPY ENDING

Every book should have a happy ending and if you are the sort of person who is always finding it a bit of a struggle to avoid putting on weight, here is one for you!

SWITCHING TO A HEALTHY DIET ENABLES US TO EAT MORE WITHOUT PUTTING ON WEIGHT!

Pork pie in the sky surely! Not at all. It depends on two simple facts. Firstly, a gram of fat contains more than twice as many calories as a gram of starch – fat yields 9kcal in a gram compared with starch's 4kcals. Secondly, as a general rule, starchy foods like potatoes are more bulky than fatty foods like butter. The result is that a pound of potatoes yields only one tenth as many calories as a pound of butter. So by cutting down on fatty foods and increasing your intake of fresh fruit and vegetables you can actually eat more without putting on weight!

THE KILOCALORIE COUNTER

Energy in the United Kingdom is measured in kilocalories. To save writing out 'kilocalories' all the time it is usually abbreviated to 'kcal' which is what you see written on food labels. In other European countries, energy is measured in Joules, which also appears on food labels, but it is too confusing to use both methods, so we are best to stick with kilocalories and forget about citizen Joules. Kilocalories is a bit of a mouthful, so people usually talk about calories, but they mean the same thing.

We obtain our energy from fat, carbohydrate and protein, and occasionally, unless we are teetotal, from alcohol. As the table below shows, fat provides over twice as many kcals as the same amount of carbohydrate or protein.

THE NUMBER OF CALORIES PROVIDED BY DIFFERENT KINDS OF FOOD

100gm (3.5oz) of fat	900 kcal
100gm (3.5oz) of carbohydrate	400 kcal
100gm (3.5oz) of protein	400 kcal
100gm (3.5oz) of alcohol	700 kcal

The amount of energy we need each day depends on our age, sex, size and how active we are, as well as on our individual metabolism. A manual worker or sportsman or sportswoman for instance will require more energy, all else being equal, than an office worker who drives to work.

The table below gives an indication of the amount of energy required by children and adults.

AVERAGE DAILY ENERGY REQUIREMENTS

Age and activity	**Males** **Kcal per day**	**Females** **Kcal per day**
Children; increases gradually with age		
1 to 3 years	1,230	1,165
4 to 6 years	1,715	1,545
7 to 10 years	1,970	1,740
11 to 14 years	2,220	1,845

15 to 18 years	2,755	2,110
Adults	**Males**	**Females**
19 to 59 years	2,550	1,920
60 to 74 years,	2,350	1,900
75 and over,	2,100	1,810

Warning: These figures are averages. Our actual energy requirements will depend on our size and individual metabolism and how active we are as well as our age.

If we consume more food than we can use the excess is stored as fat and we put on weight. It is not only the excess fat in our diet which is stored but also excess carbohydrate and protein. Although small amounts of extra carbohydrate can be stored in our liver as a kind of carbohydrate known as glycogen, the rest is converted into fat. Excess protein can also be converted into fat and stored.

As a rough guide, an active woman dashing around the aisles with her trolley, needs about 2,150 kcal a day and an active man about 2,700 kcal a little more than the average values in the table above. Even if they are the same size, women tend to use their food more efficiently, extracting more useful energy from the ounce and so need to consume less. Less active women may need no more than 1,900 kcal per day and some even less than that.

To avoid putting on weight it is obviously necessary to balance intake against activity. To reduce weight we need to consume less kcal than our daily need so that we start to draw upon our fat stores to make up the deficit.

A sure way not to lose weight permanently is to go on a crash diet for a few months and then at the end of it return to the same diet as one had at the beginning. Faced

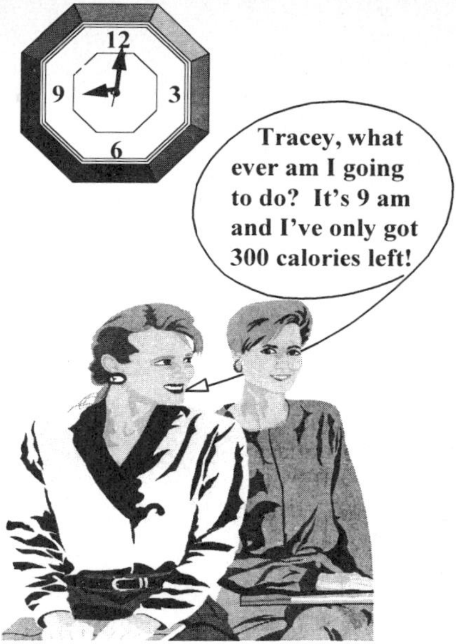

with what it thinks is a period of starvation, the body will respond as it would during a drought or other real period of food shortage by using more efficiently what little food it has coming in. Then when you stop your diet and resume eating as you did before, your body will continue to utilise the food it is getting more efficiently and store the excess as fat. By the time your body realises that the period of starvation is over, all of the fat will be back again. The only way to ensure that the fat stays off is to keep the calories down to a sensible level for evermore and to take plenty of exercise, but this can be achieved by healthy eating, with all-out dieting a thing of the past!

HOW TO USE THE SEEK AND REDUCE CALORIE AND FAT COUNTER

The Counter gives the number of calories and the amount of total fat and saturated fat in every 100 grams (3.5 oz) of each item. To give an idea of what 100g looks like, the final column tells you how many bags of crisps you need to eat, or how many biscuits and so on to obtain 100g.

Before setting off to consult the main Calorie and Fat Counter, decide what type of food you want to buy – fish, cereals, fruit and so on. To help you decide, the brief table below provides an at-a-glance guide as to roughly how many calories typical examples of different kinds of food contain.

Category of food	**Typical kcal in each 100g (3.5 oz) of ordinary product (refer to the Main Calorie Counter for diet or low fat forms of those marked with an *)**
Butter	700
Margarine	700
Nuts, without shells	600
*Crisps	550
*Biscuits	500
*Snack bars	500
*Cheese	400
*Most red meats	250-400
Breakfast cereals	350
*Cakes	350
Bread	200
Fatty fish	200
Chicken and turkey	150
White fish	100
Typical low fat yoghurts	100
Root vegetables	50

Fruit	30
Green vegetables	25

If you can't resist the high calorie foods marked with a star in the table above, be sure to seek out the low calorie, low fat options and/or cut down on the portions. So, having decided that you want to buy, say, a packet of biscuits, look up biscuits in the main Calorie and Fat Counter. Near the top of the list you will find the typical biscuits, high in calories and fat. The ones to go for are those nearest the bottom which are the lowest in fat and usually in calories as well.

If you want to lose weight, or to avoid putting it on, cut down on the fat first. Not only is too much fat, especially saturated fat, undesirable in itself, but it also contains twice as many calories per pound as starch, sugar and protein.

As you will see, most products are now available in their traditional form and as a healthy option, often manufactured by the same company. If the particular brands that I have mentioned as examples of healthier options are not stocked by your local supermarket, don't worry. They are just given as examples. Note down the fat and calorie content, and Read That Label until you find an equivalent product which is just as low in fat and calories, and go for that instead.

Even if you don't need or want to lose weight, you should still cut down on the high fat foods, and eat more high calorie, starchy foods like bread, breakfast cereals, rice, pasta and root vegetables instead to make up for the lost calories. The Calorie and Fat Counter is not, therefore, just for weight watchers, but for everyone who recognises the health benefits of a diet which is not as excessively high in saturated fat as the typical British diet tends to be. If you have a car designed to run on petrol,

The Kamikaze Pilot

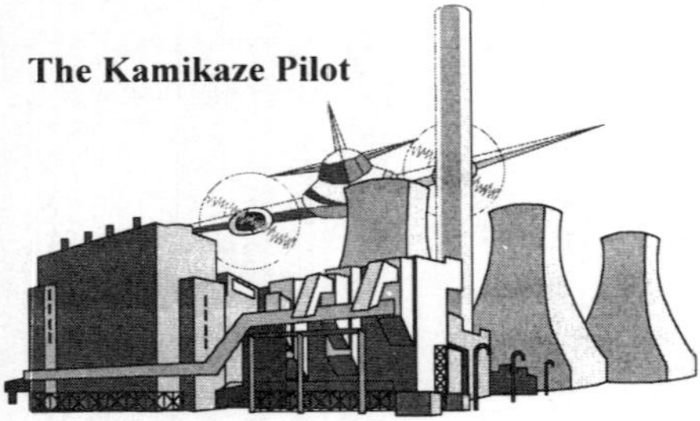

The Kamikaze Eater

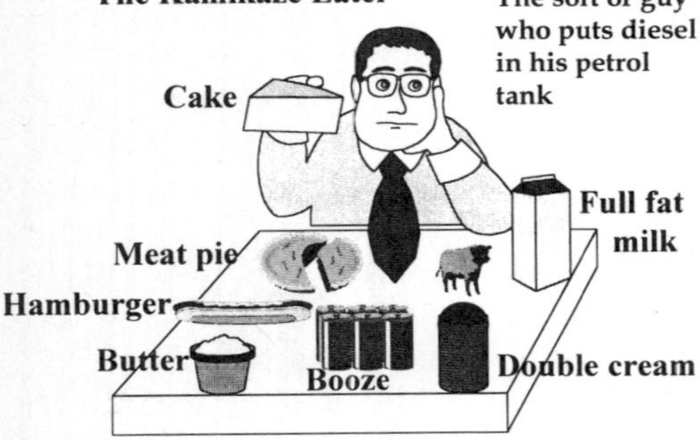

would you fill your tank with diesel? A diet high in saturated fat is not the fuel our bodies were designed to run on.

A PERSONAL ASSESSMENT OF YOUR CURRENT DIET

Would you like, by completing a simple questionnaire, to obtain a personal assessment of your current diet from the author? To find out more, send a self-addressed envelope with a first-class stamp to Dr Trevor Smith, 131 Roundhill Rd., St Andrews, Fife, Scotland, KY16 8HG.

HAPPY SUPERMARKET SHOPPING!

Product	*kcal per 100 g (3.5 oz)*	*Total fat grams per 100g*	*Saturated fat grams per 100g*	*Portions (servings, bags etc) in 100g*

Fruit

Fresh Fruit

LOW CALORIE, VIRTUALLY FAT FREE
(Weighed with skin and pips)

Apples	42	0.1		
Apricots	29	0.1		
Bananas	62	0.2		
Blackberries	25	0.2		
Blackcurrants	28	0.1		
Cherries	39	0.1		
Dates, raw	107	0.1		
Gooseberries	19	0.4		
Grapefruit	20	0.1		
Grapes	57	0.1		
Guava	24	0.5		
Kiwi fruit	42	0.4		
Lemons	19	0.3		
Lychees	36	0.1		
Mangoes	39	0.1		
Melon	16	0.1		
Nectarines	36	0.1		
Oranges	26	0.1		
Passion fruit	22	0.2		
Paw-paw	27	0.1		
Peaches	30	0.1		
Pineapple, flesh only	41	0.2		
Plum	41	0.2		
Raspberries	25	0.3		
Rhubarb	7	0.1		
Strawberries	27	0.1		
Tangerines	35	0.1		

TWO HIGH FAT EXCEPTIONS

Avocado	139	13.8	2.9	
Olives	82	8.8	1.4	

Canned Fruit

ORDINARY IN SYRUP

Peach halves, Del Monte	72	Trace		

Product	*kcal per 100 g (3.5 oz)*	*Total fat grams per 100g*	*Saturated fat grams per 100g*	*Portions (servings, bags etc) in 100g*
LOWER CALORIE IN FRUIT JUICE				
Peach halves, Del Monte	49	Trace		
Jams and Preserves				
ORDINARY				
Robertson's strawberry jam	249	Trace		
LOWER CALORIE				
Tesco, reduced sugar strawberry jam	133	Trace		

Vegetables

HIGH IN STARCH AND VITAMINS				
Beetroot	36	0.1		
Carrots	35	0.3		
Parsnips	64	1.1		
Potatoes, new	70	0.3		
Potatoes, old	75	0.2		
Radishes	12	0.2		
Swede	24	0.3		
Sweet potato	87	0.3		
Turnip	23	0.3		
Yam	114	0.3		
Green Vegetables				
LOW IN CALORIES AND FAT; HIGH IN VITAMINS				
Asparagus	25	0.6		
Aubergine	26	0.8		
Broccoli	42	1.4		
Cabbage	26	0.4		
Cauliflower	34	0.9		
Celery	7	0.2		
Chicory	11	0.6		
Courgette	18	0.4		
Cucumber	10	0.1		
Curly Kale	33	1.6		
Leeks	22	0.5		
Lettuce	14	0.5		
Marrow	12	0.2		
Mustard and Cress	13	0.6		

Product	*kcal per 100 g (3.5 oz)*	*Total fat grams per 100g*	*Saturated fat grams per 100g*	*Portions (servings, bags etc) in 100g*
Onions	36	0.2		
Peppers, green	15	0.3		
Peppers, red	32	0.4		
Pumpkin	13	0.2		
Spinach	25	0.8		
Spring onions	23	0.5		
Sweetcorn	66	1.4		
Tomatoes	17	0.3		
Watercress	22	1.0		
Peas and Beans				
EAT LOTS FOR THEIR PROTEIN				
Mange-tout peas	32	0.2		
Green beans/French beans	24	0.5		
Runner beans	22	0.4		
IN CANS (DRAINED)				
Baked beans	84	0.6		
Broad beans	81	0.6		
Butter beans	77	0.5		
Garden peas, Smedleys	49	0.3		
DRIED				
Lentils, green and brown	297	1.9		
Lentils, red, split	318	1.3		
Mung beans	279	1.1		
Red kidney beans	266	1.4		
Soya beans	370	18.6	2.3	
OTHERS				
Beansprouts	31	0.5		
Tofu, soya bean, steamed	73	4.2	0.5	
Canned Vegetables				
LOW IN CALORIES AND FAT				
For example:				
Baby carrots, Tesco	20	0.3		
Potatoes, small, new, Safeway	50	0.2		
Sweetcorn, Safeway, (unsugared)	82	0.8		

Product	*kcal per 100 g (3.5 oz)*	*Total fat grams per 100g*	*Saturated fat grams per 100g*	*Portions (servings, bags etc) in 100g*
Frozen vegetables				
LOW IN CALORIES AND FAT				
For example:				
Special mixed vegetables, Safeway	47	1.1	0.3	
Brussels sprouts, Safeway	42	1.4	0.3	
Garden peas, Bird's Eye	62	0.7	0.1	
Chips				
LOW FAT				
McCain's Oven Ready Chips	167	5.1	0.1	

Nuts

VERY HIGH IN CALORIES AND VERY HIGH IN FAT BUT IN MOST NUTS IT IS MAINLY HEALTHY UNSATURATED FAT (MEASURED WITHOUT SHELLS)

ALARMINGLY HIGH IN SATURATED FAT				
Coconuts	669	68.8	59.3	
FAIRLY HIGH IN SATURATED FAT				
Brazil nuts	682	68.2	16.4	
Cashew nuts	611	50.9	10.1	
Macadamia nuts	748	77.6	11.2	
LESS SATURATED FAT				
Almonds	612	55.8	4.7	
Hazelnuts	650	63.5	4.7	
Peanuts	564	46.1	8.2	
Pecan nuts	689	70.1	5.7	
Pistachio nuts (with shells)	331	30.5	4.1	
Walnuts	688	68.5	5.6	
EXCEPTIONALLY LOW IN CALORIES AND FAT				
Chestnuts	170	2.7	0.5	
Nut Products				
Marzipan	404	14.4	1.2	
Peanut butter	623	53.7	11.7	

Product	*kcal per 100 g (3.5 oz)*	*Total fat grams per 100g*	*Saturated fat grams per 100g*	*Portions (servings, bags etc) in 100g*
Seeds				
Sesame seeds	598	58.0	8.3	
Sunflower seeds	581	47.5	4.5	

Cereals and cereal products

FAIRLY HIGH CALORIES, BUT LOW FAT

Rice				
White, raw	383	3.6	0.9	
Brown, raw	357	2.8	0.7	
Pasta				
Spaghetti, white, raw	346	1.8	0.2	
Spaghetti, wholemeal, raw	324	2.5	0.4	
Macaroni, raw	348	1.8	0.3	
Wheat flour				
Plain white	341	1.3	0.2	
Wholemeal	310	2.2	0.3	
Bread				
White average	235	1.9	0.4	3 med. slices
Wholemeal average	215	2.5	0.5	3 med. slices
Other breads				
MUCH HIGHER IN FAT				
Chapatis, made with fat	328	12.8		
Naan bread	336	12.5		
Popadums, fried in vegetable oil	369	16.9	1.7	

Breakfast cereals

FAIRLY HIGH CALORIES, BUT LOW SATURATED FAT

All-Bran	261	3.4		
Bran Flakes	318	1.9		
Coco Pops	384	1.0		
Common Sense	357	4.0		
Corn Flakes	360	0.7		
Crunchy Nut Corn Flakes	398	4.0		

Product	*kcal per 100 g (3.5 oz)*	*Total fat grams per 100g*	*Saturated fat grams per 100g*	*Portions (servings, bags etc) in 100g*
Frosties	377	0.5		
Fruit 'n' Fibre	349	4.7		
Muesli, Swiss style	363	5.9		
Oat and Wheat Bran	325	3.5		
Porridge	49	1.1		
Puffed Wheat	328	1.3		
Raisin Splitz	337	2.0		
Ready Brek	373	7.8		
Rice Krispies	369	0.9		
Ricicles	381	0.5		
Shredded Wheat, Nestlé	352	2.2		
Shreddies	331	1.5		
Smacks	386	2.0		
Special K	377	1.0		
Sugar Puffs	348	0.8		
Sultana Bran	303	1.6		
Weetabix	352	2.7		
Weetaflake	359	2.8		
Weetos	372	2.7		

Biscuits

TYPICAL BISCUITS HAVE TWICE AS MANY CALORIES AS BREAD; THEY ALSO HAVE TEN TIMES AS MUCH FAT, HALF OF IT SATURATED

Digestive biscuits

A 300G PACKET OF ORDINARY DIGESTIVES HAS OVER HALF AS MANY CALORIES AS WE NEED IN A DAY, SO YOU SEE HOW FATTENING THEY ARE!

ORDINARY

Chocolate				
McVitie's chocolate wholewheat	506	24.0	12.1	6 biscuits
Spar, chocolate	511	24.2		8 biscuits
Plain				
McVities's standard	495	21.9	9.9	7 biscuits

Product	*kcal per 100 g (3.5 oz)*	*Total fat grams per 100g*	*Saturated fat grams per 100g*	*Portions (servings, bags etc) in 100g*
LOWER FAT				
McVitie's light , 25% less fat	467	16.4	7.2	7 biscuits
Burton's Trim half fat	420	11.5	4.7	7 biscuits
Other Kinds of Biscuit				
ORDINARY				
Shortbread	498	26.1		
Oatcakes	441	18.3		
Gingernut biscuits	456	15.2		
Cream crackers	418	14.5		12 biscuits
LOWER FAT				
Crispbread	321			
Wholemeal crackers	413	11.3		
Jaffa cakes, McVitie's	376	8.2		
Cream Crackers, Jacob's Light	400	7.1		12 biscuits
Burton's Rich Tea, half fat	404	6.2	2.5	10 biscuits

Cakes and Puddings

A TYPICAL CAKE HAS HALF AS MANY CALORIES AGAIN AS BREAD, IT ALSO HAS FIVE TO TEN TIMES AS MUCH FAT

Chocolate Gateau				
ORDINARY				
Cadbury's Chocolate Gateau	320	20.8		
Rich chocolate gateau, Marks and Spencer's	342	18.7	9.0	
LOWER FAT				
Safeway Orange and Chocolate Gateau	218	5.5	3.6	
Other Kinds of Cake				
ORDINARY				
Battenburg cake, Mr Kipling	380	9.9		
Fancy iced cakes (average)	407	14.9		
Fruit cake, plain	354	12.9		
rich iced	356	11.4		
Madeira cake, Mr Kipling	325	14.5		
Swiss rolls (average)	337	11.3		
Scones, fruit	316	9.8		
plain	362	14.6		
wholemeal	326	14.4		

Product	*kcal per 100 g (3.5 oz)*	*Total fat grams per 100g*	*Saturated fat grams per 100g*	*Portions (servings, bags etc) in 100g*
Scotch pancakes	273	17.5		
Teacakes, Tunnock's	413	18.1		
Cake bars				
Flapjacks, apricot & raisin, Mr Kipling	438	22.9		3 cakes
Jaffa cake bar, McVitie's	408	16.9		3 bars
Golden syrup cake bars, McVitie's	376	11.8		3 cakes
LOWER FAT				
Chocolate Arctic Roll, Blue Ribbon, Wall's	225	6.9	4.9	2 X 50g servings
Cakes with Fruit & Nuts, Mr Kipling	118	5.4		
Sponge cake, jam filled (average)	302	4.9		
Buns and Pastries				
ORDINARY				
Jam tarts, Mr Kipling	386	14.5		3 tarts
Jam tarts, Safeway	393	15.4		3 tarts
Mince pies	423	20.4		
Fruit pie, individual (average)	369	15.5		
Lemon meringue pie	319	14.4		
Apple pies, Lyon's	369	15.0		
Safeway's Bramley	393	12.7	3.4	
LOWER FAT				
Apple pie, McVitie's	235	9.6		
Hot cross buns	310	6.8		
Puddings and Fruit Pies				
ORDINARY HIGH FAT				
Typical sponge pudding	340	16.3		
Treacle tart	368	14.1		
Peach and apricot tart, Marks and Spencer's.	220	9.6	4.7	
LOW FAT				

Product	*kcal per 100 g (3.5 oz)*	*Total fat grams per 100g*	*Saturated fat grams per 100g*	*Portions (servings, bags etc) in 100g*
Ambrosia creamed rice	90	1.6		
Ambrosia low fat rice puddings	76	0.8	0.4	

Crisps

ORDINARY CRISPS ARE AS HIGH IN FAT AS BACON. THEY ARE ALSO HIGH IN CALORIES. BEWARE THE DIFFERENT SIZED BAGS!

ORDINARY				
Typical standard potato crisps (average of 20 types)	546	37.6	9.2	
KP crisps, salted	545	36.8		4 bags
Quavers, Walker's	564	37.5		6 bags
Cheese and onion crisps, Walker's,	550	38.0		3 bags
Potato rings, Safeway	538	33.0	15.2	1.3 bags
A SINGLE 75G PACKET INFLICTS 11G SATURATED FAT!				
Crisps, KP	525	33.3	8.7	4 bags
Brannigans thick cut potato crisps, KP	507	30.3		3 bags
Idaho chips, Royster's	516	31.5	8.2	4 bags
LOW IN SATURATED FAT				
Highlander crisps	500	35.7	4.3	3 bags
ONE THIRD LOWER IN TOTAL FAT BUT BEWARE THE BIG BAGS!				
Low fat cheese and onion crisps, Tesco	471	24.8	11.4	1.5 bags
Reduced fat crinkles, Marks & Spencer's	474	24	10.7	1.5 bags
BUY SENSIBLE-SIZED BAGS				
Golden Lights, Golden Wonder	457	20		3 bags
Solos Lites, KP	469	22.8	9.8	4.5 bags

AIM FOR SNACKS WITH MUCH LOWER TOTAL FAT AND CALORIE LEVELS LIKE:

Reduced fat, bacon hoops, potato snack, Boots	399	12	6	3 bags

Product	*kcal per 100 g (3.5 oz)*	*Total fat grams per 100g*	*Saturated fat grams per 100g*	*Portions (servings, bags etc) in 100g*
Potato Crisp Waffles, The Low Fat Snack Company	329	1		3 bags

Corn and Other Snacks

ORDINARY

Corn snacks (average of 20 different types)	519	31.9	11.8	

LOW IN SATURATED FAT, BUT AGAIN BEWARE OF BIG BAGS!

Pizza bread snacks, Tesco	519	27.6	4.2	1 bag
Tortilla chips (average of 6 brands)	459	22	4.0	
Golden Onion Rings, Marks and Spencer's	483	19.4	3.5	2 bags

MUCH LOWER IN TOTAL FAT

Pasta twists, Safeway	425	14.7	2.9	
Twiglets, Jacobs	401	12.8		1 bag with 100 twiglets
Garlic flavour breadsticks, Tesco	407	7.8	1.1	20 sticks

Dairy Products

Milk

Full fat	60	3.9	2.4	About 2/5
Semi-skimmed	49	1.7	1.0	mug
Skimmed	34	0.1		

Cheese

ALWAYS GO FOR THE HALF FAT CHEESE: JUST AS MUCH PROTEIN AND CALCIUM AS FULL FAT

ORDINARY

White Cheddar	410	34.4	21.7	
Red Leicester	399	33.7	21.1	

HALF FAT, LOWER CALORIES

Shape half fat Cheddar, St Ivel	259	16.5	10.4	
Shape half fat Red Leicester	262	16.1	10.1	

COTTAGE

Shape, virtually fat free	67	0.2	0.1	

Product	*kcal per 100 g (3.5 oz)*	*Total fat grams per 100g*	*Saturated fat grams per 100g*	*Portions (servings, bags etc) in 100g*
Cheese spreads				
GO FOR THE HALF-FAT AND LOWER VARIETIES				
ORDINARY				
Dairylea Regular, Kraft	285	23.5	15.5	4 triangles
HALF FAT, LOWER CALORIES				
Cheddarie Light, Kraft	240	15.0	10.0	
Philadelphia low fat cheese spread,Kraft	187	15.0	10.0	
Dairylea Light, Kraft	185	11.0	7.3	
Delight, low fat dairy spread	181	10.0	6.0	
Margarine				
ORDINARY				
Stork golden	731	81	34	
Vitalite, sunflower spread	637	70	16	
LOWER FAT, LOWER CALORIES				
Vitalite, light	352	52	10	
Flora Extra Light (only 0.4g trans-fatty acids)	368	39	9	
Ice cream				
ORDINARY				
Choc-ices				
Feast, Wall's	329	24.1		
Plain ice-cream				
Vanilla Soft Scoop, Safeway	178	7.8	7.3	2 scoops
Vanilla Flavour Ice Cream, Safeway	154	7.0	3.3	
Mini milk ice lollies, Wall's	112	3.4		3 lollies
VERY LOW FAT, LOWER CALORIE				
Virtually fat free, vanilla flavour frozen dessert, Safeway	112	0.4	"	
Too Good To Be True, Wall's	93	0.4	"	
Yogurt				
HIGH FAT AND HIGH CALORIES				
Greek, Safeway	128	10.0	6.4	

Product	*kcal per 100 g (3.5 oz)*	*Total fat grams per 100g*	*Saturated fat grams per 100g*	*Portions (servings, bags etc) in 100g*
LOW FAT				
Dozens of brands available e.g.:				
Low Fat Yoghurt, Hazelnut, Asda (19.6g sugar)	115	1.7	0.8	two-thirds of a pot
Ski, extra fruit, strawberry and melon	100	1.0		
VERY LOW FAT AND LOW CALORIES				
Very Low Fat, Light natural Yoghurt,Asda (9.7g sugar)	67	0.2		two-thirds of a pot
Very Low Fat Light Yogurt, raspberry and vanilla, Asda (6.2g sugar)	44	0.1		2 pots
Muller Light,Very Low Fat Yogurt	49	0.1		Half a 200g pot
Fromage Frais, Tesco	46	0.2		
Chocolate Mousse				
ORDINARY WITH VERY HIGH FAT				
Aero Milk Chocolate Mousse, Nestlé	230	13.2	6.9	
Dairy Milk Mousse, Cadbury's	232	11.3		
LOWER FAT				
Low fat chocolate mousse, Cadbury's light	123	4.7		

Meat and Poultry

CAREFULLY REMOVING ALL OF THE VISIBLE FAT CAN REDUCE THE FAT CONTENT OF MEAT BY A HALF AND CALORIES BY A THIRD. MUCH OF THE VISIBLE FAT IS UNDESIRABLE SATURATED FAT.

Lamb

GO FOR THE LEANER CUTS AND REMOVE VISIBLE FAT

Breast, roast	410	37.1	14.3
Cutlets, grilled	370	30.9	15.3
Loin chops, grilled	355	29.0	14.4
Shoulder, roast	316	26.3	13.1

Product	*kcal per 100 g (3.5 oz)*	*Total fat grams per 100g*	*Saturated fat grams per 100g*	*Portions (servings, bags etc) in 100g*
Scrag & neck, stewed	292	21.1	10.5	
Leg, roast	266	17.9	8.9	
Breast, roast, with visible fat removed	252	16.6	6.2	
Beef				
GO FOR THE LEANER CUTS AND REMOVE VISIBLE FAT				
Brisket, boiled	26	23.9	9.5	
Forerib, roast	349	28.8	12.3	
Sirloin, roast	284	21.1	9.0	
Mince, stewed	229	15.2	6.5	
Rump steak, fried	246	14.6	6.2	
Silverside, boiled	242	14.2	6.2	
Rump steak, grilled	218	12.1	5.2	
Topside, roast	214	12.0	4.1	
Stewing steak, stewed	223	11.0	4.7	
Pork				
Belly rashers, grilled	398	34.8	12.9	
Leg, roast	286	19.8	7.3	
Trotters and tails, boiled	280	22.3		
Loin chops, with visible fat removed, grilled	226	10.7	3.8	
Bacon				
VERY HIGH IN FAT AND CALORIES. REMOVE ALL VISIBLE FAT				
Streaky, fried	496	44.8	17.5	
Middle, fried	477	42.3	16.5	
Back, fried	465	40.6	15.9	
Streaky, grilled	422	36.0	14.1	
Middle, grilled	416	35.1	13.8	
Collar joint, boiled	325	27.0	10.6	
Rashers, lean fried	332	22.3	8.3	
Rashers, lean grilled	292	18.9	7.4	
Gammon, boiled	269	18.9	7.4	
Raw Kidney				
Lamb, ox and pig average	90	2.7	1.0	
Raw Liver				

Product	*kcal per 100 g (3.5 oz)*	*Total fat grams per 100g*	*Saturated fat grams per 100g*	*Portions (servings, bags etc) in 100g*
Calf, lamb, ox and pig average	162	8.1	2.5	
Lamb's tongue				
Raw	193	14.6		
Wild Game				
LOW IN FAT AND CALORIES				
Roast Venison	198	6.4		
Rabbit				
Raw, meat only	124	4.0	1.6	
Stewed, meat only	179	7.7	3.2	
Roast Chicken				
BECAUSE POULTRY IS LOWER IN FAT, IT IS ALSO LOWER IN CALORIES THAN RED MEAT. REMOVE THE SKIN TO GET RID OF MOST OF THE FAT				
Meat and skin	216	14.0	4.2	
Meat only	148	5.4	1.6	
Dark meat	155	6.9	2.1	
Light meat	142	4.0	1.2	
Leg quarter, meat only	92	3.4	1.0	
Wing quarter, meat only	74	2.7	0.8	
Roast Turkey				
TURKEY IS THE LEANEST MEAT AROUND. TO MAKE IT EVEN LEANER, REMOVE THE SKIN				
Meat and skin	171	6.5	2.1	
Meat only	140	2.7	0.9	
Dark meat	148	4.1	1.3	
Light meat	132	1.4	0.4	
Roast Pheasant				
FAIRLY LEAN				
Meat only	213	9.3	3.1	
Roast Pigeon				
FAIRLY LEAN				
Meat only	230	13.2		

Product	*kcal per 100 g (3.5 oz)*	*Total fat grams per 100g*	*Saturated fat grams per 100g*	*Portions (servings, bags etc) in 100g*
Roast Duck				
A LOT OF FAT IN THE SKIN				
Meat, fat and skin	339	29.0	7.9	
Meat only	189	9.7	2.7	
Roast Goose				
A LOT OF FAT				
Meat only	319	22.4		
Meat Products				
ALMOST ALL MEAT PRODUCTS ARE VERY HIGH IN FAT				
Beefburgers, raw	265	20.5	9.5	
Black pudding	305	21.9	8.5	
Cornish pastie	332	20.4	7.4	
Faggots	268	18.5		
Frankfurters	274	25.0		
Haggis	310	21.7	7.6	
Sausage roll	477	36.4	13.4	
Pork pie	376	27.0	10.2	
Steak and kidney pie	323	21.2	8.4	
Meat paste	173	11.2		
Sausages and Paté				
VERY HIGH IN FAT				
Salami	491	45.2		
Pate	316	28.9	8.4	
Pork sausages	367	32.1	12.2	
Beef sausages	299	24.1	10.0	
LOWER FAT				
Low fat sausages	166	9.5	3.4	
Canned Meat				
Ham and pork, chopped, canned	275	23.6		
Luncheon meat, canned	313	26.9		
Corned beef, Princes'	216	12.8		
Corned beef, Fray Bentos	209	11.6		
LOWER FAT				
Ham, Ye Olde Oak, Reformed	108	5.5		

Product	*kcal per 100 g (3.5 oz)*	*Total fat grams per 100g*	*Saturated fat grams per 100g*	*Portions (servings, bags etc) in 100g*
FISH				
White Fish				
HIGH IN PROTEIN, LOW IN CALORIES AND FAT				
(Measured raw)				
Cod	76	0.7	0.1	
Haddock	73	0.6	0.1	
Halibut	92	2.4	0.3	
Lemon sole	81	1.4	0.2	
Plaice	91	2.2	0.3	
Saithe	73	0.5	0.1	
Whiting, steamed	92	0.9	0.1	
Fatty Fish				
TWICE AS HIGH IN CALORIES AS WHITE FISH BUT RICH IN ESSENTIAL FATTY ACIDS				
Herring, raw	234	18.5	5.3	
Kipper, baked with bones	111	6.2	1.0	
Mackerel	223	16.3	3.3	
Salmon	182	12.0	2.2	
Trout, steamed	89	3.0	0.7	
Canned				
Pilchards in tomato sauce	126	5.4	1.1	
Sardines in oil (drained)	217	13.6	2.8	
Sardines in tomato sauce (drained)	177	11.6	3.3	
Tuna in oil (drained)	189	9.0	1.4	
Tuna in brine (drained)	99	0.6	0.2	
Fish Products				
HIGH IN FAT				
Cod in batter, fried in oil, fish & chip shops	199	10.3	0.9	
fried in dripping	199	10.3	4.7	
Fish fingers, fried in blended oil (average of 3 brands)	233	12.7	2.8	
Fish paste (average of 30 samples)	169	10.4		
Roe, cod, hard, fried	202	11.9	1.2	
Roe, herring, soft, fried	244	15.8	1.6	

Product	*kcal per 100 g (3.5 oz)*	*Total fat grams per 100g*	*Saturated fat grams per 100g*	*Portions (servings, bags etc) in 100g*
Crustacea				
LOW IN CALORIES AND FAT				
Crab, boiled with shell	25	1.0	0.1	
Lobster, boiled with shell	42	1.2		
Prawns, boiled with shell	41	0.7	0.2	
Shrimps, frozen, shell removed	73	0.8	0.1	
Molluscs				
LOW IN CALORIES AND FAT				
Cockles, boiled	48	0.3	0.1	
Mussels, boiled with shell	26	0.6	0.1	
Squid, frozen, raw	66	1.5		
Whelks, boiled with shell	14	0.3	0.1	
Winkles, boiled with shell	14	0.3		

Confectionery

Chocolate bars				
AS HIGH IN FAT AS PORK VERY HIGH IN CALORIES				
ORDINARY				
Milkybar Buttons, Nestlé	549	32.5		
Twirl, Cadbury's	525	30.1		
Dairy Milk Chocolate, Cadbury's	525	29.4		
Flake, Cadbury's	505	28.5		
KitKat, Nestlé Rowntree	502	26.0	2 bars (48g)	
Twix, Mars	495	24.2		
A THIRD LESS FAT BUT STILL HIGH IN CALORIES				
Crunchy, Cadbury's	490	18.8		
Mars	452	17.5	10	1.5 bars (65g)
Milky Way, Mars	454	16.6	8	
Light Nougat Crisp, Boots	369	14	10	3 bars (30g)
VERY LOW IN SATURATED FAT				
Frusli, Jordans	431	17.1	3.4	3 bars (33g)

Product	*kcal per 100 g (3.5 oz)*	*Total fat grams per 100g*	*Saturated fat grams per 100g*	*Portions (servings, bags etc) in 100g*

Drinks

(Amounts are per 100 ml)

THE CALORIES DEPEND ON HOW MUCH YOU DRINK: A MEDIUM SIZED MUG WOULD HOLD ABOUT 250 ML, SO MULTIPLY THE KCALS IN 100 ML BY TWO AND A HALF

Pure Fruit Juice

NO ARTIFICIAL PRESERVATIVES, COLOURS OR FLAVOURINGS. A GOOD HEALTHY SOURCE OF CALORIES.

Orange juice	45	Nil		
Orange and pineapple juice, Safeway	42	Nil		
Carrot juice, organic, Eden	28	Nil		
Tomato juice, Del Monte	24	Nil		
Sparkling white grape juice, Safeway	60	Nil		

Fruit Juice Drinks

ORDINARY

Ribena blackcurrant	60	Nil		
Cranberry classic, Ocean Spray	49	Nil		
Bitter lemon, Safeway	32	Nil		

DIET (In diet varieties added sugar is replaced by artificial sweetener)

Ribena blackcurrant, light	22	Nil		
Bitter lemon, Schweppes, slimline	2	Nil		

Fizzy drinks

Lucozade	76	Nil		
Ginger Ale, Sunrise (contains artificial sweeteners)	22	Nil		
Sparkling lemonade, Safeway	25	Nil		

Diet Fizzy Drinks

WITH COLOURINGS AND PRESERVATIVES

For example:

Irn Bru	4			
Tango	4			

Product	*kcal per 100 g (3.5 oz)*	*Total fat grams per 100g*	*Saturated fat grams per 100g*	*Portions (servings, bags etc) in 100g*
NO COLOURINGS OR PRESERVATIVES				
For example:				
Diet 7-UP (but contains artificial sweeteners)	1.7			
Diet Coke (but contains artificial sweeteners)	0.4			
Squashes (diluted 1 in 4)				
Lifestyle whole orange drink (contains artificial sweeteners)	*10*			
Alcoholic Drinks				(kcal in a pint)
BEERS				
Strong ale	72			409
Beer	32			182
Lager	29			165
Low alcohol beers and lagers	20			114
CIDERS				
Sweet cider	42			239
Dry cider	36			205
WINES				(kcal in a 140 ml glass)
Rosé wine	71			99
Red wine	68			95
Sweet white wine	94			132
Dry white wine	66			92
FORTIFIED WINES				(kcal in a 50 ml glass)
Port	157			79
Sweet sherry	136			68
Dry sherry	116			58
VERMOUTH				
Sweet	151			76
Dry	118			59
LIQUEURS				(kcal in a 25 ml glass)
Advocaat	272			68
Cherry brandy	255			64
SPIRITS	200			50

Ready Made Meals

There are so many and varied that the only answer is to read the label. Just a few examples to give an idea of the variation in fat content between different meals and different brands of the same meal. Remember, a serving is about 250gm and the figures given are per 100gm, so you will need to multiply by two and a half to get an idea of how many calories and how much fat you will consume at a meal.

Product	*kcal per 100 g (3.5 oz)*	*Total fat grams per 100g*	*Saturated fat grams per 100g*	*Portions (servings, bags etc) in 100g*
HIGH CALORIES, HIGH FAT				
Macaroni Cheese, Marks and Spencer's	191	10.3	6.0	
MEDIUM CALORIES, MEDIUM FAT				
Macaroni Cheese, Safeway	122	4.5	2.7	
Chicken breast roast (with sausages and stuffing), Marks and Spencer's	149	7.7	2.1	
Haddock & Chips (and peas), Marks and Spencer's	161	6.1	1.0	
Lasagne, Safeway	119	4.8	2.9	
LOW CALORIES, LOW FAT				
Glazed chicken, Birds Eye Healthy Options	89	2.5	0.6	
Beef goulash, Heinz Weight Watchers	91	2.0	0.6	
Prawn currie and rice, Findus	95	2.6	0.9	
Haddock and cauliflower cheese, Lite, Marks and Spencer's	70	1.7	1.0	
Fresh vegetable ratatouille, M & S	50	3.1	0.6	

Sources of Data and Further Reading

The reports on which the main recommendations in this book are based

Nutritional Aspects of Cardiovascular Disease. Report of the Cardiovascular Review Group Committee on Medical Aspects of Food Policy (COMA), Report on Health and Social Subjects No 46, published by HMSO for the Department of health in 1944. Price £10. (ISBN 0 11 321875 3). A must for all professional nutritionists, but the casual reader might find it a bit of a slog.

The Scottish Diet. Report of a working Party for the Chief Medical Officer for Scotland. Published by Scottish Home and Health Department in 1993. (ISBN 0748 007 970). Makes straightforward recommendations based on the available evidence but otherwise is again a bit heavy going for the casual reader.

Welfare of farm animals

The Kind Food Guide, by Audrey Eyton, published by Penguin in 1991 at £3.99. Extremely readable and informative. A must for everyone who wants to know about the lifestyle of the farm animals they are eating.

Additives

E for additives, by Maurice Hanssen, published by Thorsons Publishers Ltd. This is the long established basic guide, but pocket booklets on the subject are also available at supermarket checkouts.

Food Composition

For a more detailed calorie and fat counter there are:

Collins Gem Calorie Counter, published by Harper Collins in 1995 at £2.99.

This gives the calories and fat etc. per 100 gram of product.

Slimmer Magazine Guide to Calories and Fat, compiled and edited by Tanya May. Published by Turret Group plc, Summer 1995 at £1.75.

This gives most of the values in portions of the food rather than per 100 gram.

McCance and Widdowson's *The Composition of Foods*, 5th Edition, published by the Royal Society of Chemistry and Ministry of Agriculture, Fisheries and Food in 1991. This is the original source of the data on the calorie and nutrient content of basic foodstuffs in the other calorie counters and books on nutrition including this guide. Expensive at around £30, but it gives vitamin, mineral and cholesterol levels etc. as well as those of calories and fats. Software suitable for use by dieticians is also available from the Royal Society of Chemistry.

Manual of Nutrition. An abbreviated form of McCance and Widdowson's from the Ministry of Agriculture, Fisheries and Food. Published by HMSO, 1995 at £5.95. Highly recommended.

Exercise

Fitness Walking, by Les Snowdon and Maggie Humphreys, published by Mainstream in 1992. Useful ideas on how to build up your fitness by a programme of brisk walking. That's the best way to start, then once you are fit, you can progress on to jogging and more strenuous activities if you wish.

General

Food sense; food safety; additives; food protection; healthy eating; the new microwave labels; pesticides; monitoring our food and nutrition; radioactivity in food; natural toxicants in our food; food emergencies; keeping food cool and safe; food allergy and other unpleasant reactions to food; chemicals in food, managing the risks. All of these booklets are available, free of charge, from: Food sense, London, SE99 7TT.

Which way to health?, published quarterly by the Consumers' Association. Lots of up to date food news. Well worth subscribing to.

Food Watch, Drew Smith, published by Harper Collins in 1994 at £9.99. Gives interesting information on a variety of foods familiar and not so familiar. By dipping into it you can obtain lots of ideas on new things to try, but you will usually need to look elsewhere to find out if they are healthy or not.

The Stone-Age Health Programme, by S Boyd Eaton, Marjorie Shostak and Melvin Konner, published by Angus and Robertson Publishers in 1988 at £4.95. Don't be put off by the corny title; it is one of the best books on diet around. It demonstrates just how far today's high fat, high salt western diet has diverged from what the human body evolved over millions of years to handle.

Nutrition in General Practice, edited by Judith Buttriss. Published in 1994 by the Royal Society of General Practitioners, and available from them at 14 Princes Gate, Hyde Park, London, SW7 1PU. (ISBN 0 0584 195 X.) A guide for general practitioners on what constitutes a healthy diet and how to help their patients adopt one. Written in plain English and suitable for a wider audience than GPs alone.

Data

Data from The Composition of Foods are reproduced with the permission of The Royal Society of Chemistry and the Controller of Her Majesty's Stationery Office.

Index